Choices Coach

Weight Loss Menu Guide

Sara Moser

Although the author and publisher have made every effort to ensure that the information in this book was correct at press time, the author and publisher do not assume and hereby disclaim any liability to any party for any loss, damage, or disruption caused by errors or omissions, whether such errors or omissions result from negligence, accident, or any other cause. All the nutrition facts and menu items were taken from company web sites over the course of 2011 to 2015. Over the course of time restaurants may change their menu items and corresponding nutrition facts. In addition, the calorie content of a meal can vary depending on the consistency in preparation. Also it is worth noting that the Food and Drug Administration allows for calories on nutrition labels to be rounded.

This program is intended for healthy adults, age 18 and over. This book is solely informational and is not medical advice, nor is it intended as a substitute for the medical advice of physicians. The reader should regularly consult a physician in matters relating to his/her health and particularly with respect to any symptoms that may require diagnosis or medical attention. This book does not supersede any advice from your physician. You should check with your physician before embarking on any weight loss, diet, or exercise regimen.

Consuming raw or undercooked meats, poultry, seafood, shellfish, or eggs may increase your risk of food-borne illness, especially if you have certain medical conditions.

ISBN-13: 978-1505856897
ISBN-10: 1505856892

This book is dedicated to Danny Tinsley, the wonderful man who encouraged me to finish this book.

Contents

Introduction

I love food. I have been a personal trainer since 2007. Before I became a trainer I was overweight. I would love to tell you that after I became a trainer it was easy to stay thin from there on out. That simply was not the case. Over the past six years my weight has fluctuated. I would get tired of counting calories. I would fall off the wagon and eat/drink my calories with reckless abandon.

At the beginning of 2014, I was overweight again. Over the course of a year I lost approximately 30-35 pounds through diet and exercise. While calorie counting played a vital role in my weight loss journey I cannot tell you that I tracked my calories religiously. Even though calorie counting works it is difficult to continue on a long-term basis.

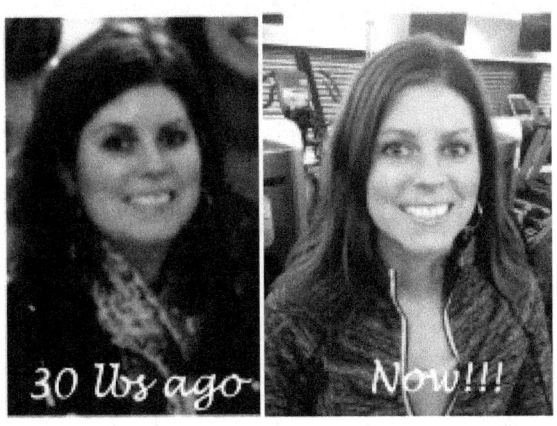

30 lbs ago   Now!!!

I have trained several clients that struggle with the same issue. They become overwhelmed with counting calories or points. Tracking a few days seems tolerable until life gets busy. The task becomes tedious, daunting, or forgotten.

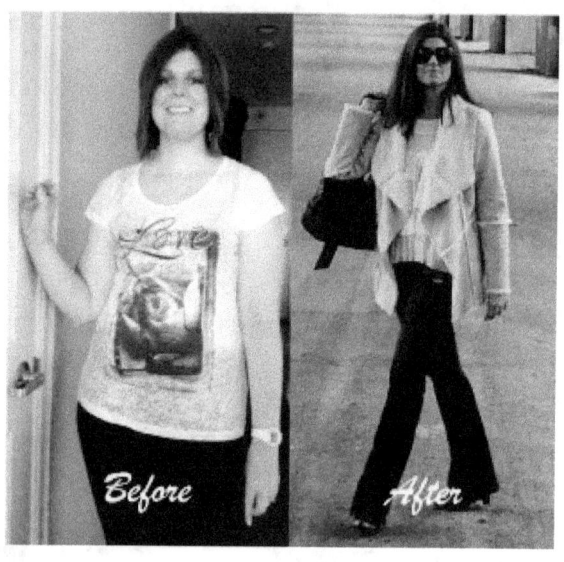

I have written this book to make calorie counting less of an issue. The book can be used as a tool to plan your meals. Imagine that this book is your selected menu when dining out. The key is to plan ahead and make healthier choices. I recommend planning three meals per day plus one or two snacks. If you are trying to lose weight, then limit yourself to one snack until you reach your goal weight. If you are working out vigorously, then definitely add the second snack to keep up your energy.

How does it work? There is a calorie budget set for each meal of the day. Then I have supplied several meal choices that fall within that budget. The budget is as follows:

Breakfast 200 to 400 calories
Lunch 300 to 500 calories
Snacks 150 calories
Dinner 550 to 650 calories

If you plan out 3 meals plus a snack, then you will be falling somewhere between 1200 to 1700 calories. If you add an additional snack, then you will be consuming approximately 1350 to 1850 calories. Please consult with your physician or dietitian regarding the appropriate calorie target for you to reach your goals.

In order to measure your portions you will need a few tools. You will need a set of both dry and liquid measuring cups, measuring spoons, and a digital food scale. I recommend purchasing a digital food scale that can toggle from grams to ounces.

This book is not an all-inclusive calorie counter, and it is not necessarily a plan to get ripped. It is simply a tool to make lower calorie choices on a daily basis in a very realistic, easy way. Once you have your calories under control, then take it a step further. Eliminate excess fat and sugar from your diet. I would be remiss if I didn't tell you that excess saturated fat and excess sugar wreak havoc on your metabolism. I have no desire to replicate the books that are already out there that cover the subject at length.

Fresh whole food is certainly better for you, so why did I include so many restaurants? I have covered fast food and sit-down dining, because it is a reality in American culture. I am not suggesting that you eat out all the time. We all know it is easier to eat healthy at home. However, that knowledge is not stopping countless people from eating out. It is a reality that dining out is social, convenient, and often fun. That is pretty tough to give up.

Several meal plans are hard to stick with, because they are too rigid. They might be healthy, but everyone's palate is different. If a meal plan includes a lot of foods that you do not enjoy, then you probably will not stick with it very long.

My ultimate goal with this book was to answer the question, "What can I eat?" It is a lot more fun to talk about what we can eat than what not to eat. There is a lot of variety. You should be able to find options that you enjoy. I recommend keeping a hard copy of the book in your handbag, brief case, or the glove compartment of your vehicle so that it is handy when you need it to make good choices.

Breakfast

For Breakfast I recommend staying within a range of 200 to 400 calories. I am sure you have probably heard that breakfast is the most important meal of the day. That doesn't mean that it has to be a huge meal, especially if you are not that hungry first thing in the morning. If you start the day with a 200 calorie breakfast, then you can certainly afford to have a mid-morning snack within your calorie budget. Be aware of your calories on beverages. They can really add up in juices, whole milk, and high-calorie coffee drinks. Start the day with water, and drink a minimum of 64 ounces throughout the day.

Coffee is a beverage that seems to polarize people. Most people either love it or hate it. As a trainer I acquired a taste for it, because it was the only way I could get up on time for a 5:30 a.m. appointment with a smile on my face. Because of my own bias plus the popularity of the beverage I have included coffee in the majority of the breakfast meal plans. If you are not a coffee drinker don't worry. You may sub in another beverage of similar calories:

Unsweetened Green Tea 0 (Top Pick!)
Coffee with 2 Tbsp. Half & Half 40
Coffee with 1 Tbsp. Non-Dairy Flavored Creamer 35
Coffee with 2 Tbsp. Non-Dairy Flavored Creamer 70
8 oz. Skim Milk 90

8 oz. 1% Milk 105
8 oz. 2% Milk 120
4.5 oz. Chocolate Skim Milk 90
8 oz. Original Soy Milk Light 60
8 oz. Vanilla Soy Milk Light 70
8 oz. Chocolate Soy Milk Light 90
8 oz. Original Pure Coconut Milk 80
8 oz. Original Almond Milk 60
8 oz. Unsweetened Vanilla Almond Milk 40
8 oz. Vanilla Almond Milk 90
8 oz. Chocolate Almond Milk 90
8 oz. Orange Juice Light 50
4 oz. Orange Juice 55
8 oz. POM Pomegranate Juice Light 75
8 oz. Big Train Fit Frappe Protein Drink, prepared or
1 Scoop (Assorted Flavors) 60 - 70
8.25 oz. Muscle Milk Light (Assorted Flavors, Lactose Free) 100
11 oz. EAS AdvantEdge Carb Control Shake (Assorted Flavors) 110

Breakfast Fast Food

Burger King

Quaker Oatmeal Original 140
Small Iced Coffee 80
Total Calories 220

Quaker Oatmeal Maple and Brown Sugar 270
Small Iced Coffee 80
Total Calories 350

Sausage Burrito 290
Small Iced Coffee 80
Total Calories 370

Breakfast Muffin Sandwich: Egg and Cheese 220
Small Iced Coffee 80
Total Calories 300

Breakfast Muffin Sandwich: Ham, Egg, and Cheese 260
Small Iced Coffee 80
Total Calories 340

Breakfast Muffin Sandwich: Bacon, Egg, and Cheese 250
Small Iced Coffee 80
Total Calories 330

3 French Toast Sticks 224
1 oz. syrup 120
Coffee with 2 creamers 46
Total Calories 390

Egg & Cheese Crossan'wich 300
Coffee with 2 creamers 46
Total Calories 346

Dunkin' Donuts

Egg White & Cheese Wheat Muffin 250
Vanilla Iced Latte Lite 90
Total Calories 340

Egg & Cheese Wake-Up Wrap 180
Vanilla Iced Latte Lite 90
Total Calories 270

Bacon Egg White & Cheese Wheat Muffin 290
Vanilla Iced Latte Lite 90
Total Calories 380

Bacon Egg & Cheese Wake-up Wrap 210
Vanilla Iced Latte Lite 90
Total Calories 300

Egg White Veggie Flatbread 330
Vanilla Iced Latte Lite 90
Total Calories 420

Glazed Munchkin 70
Vanilla Iced Latte Lite 90
Total Calories 160

Einstein Brothers

Turkey Sausage Egg White Salsa Sandwich Thin 230
16 oz. Iced Nonfat Latte 90
Total Calories 320

Egg White Asparagus and Mushroom Thin 280
12 oz. Nonfat Cappuccino 90
Total Calories 370

Fruit & Yogurt Parfait 230
12 oz. Nonfat Cafe Latte 100
Total Calories 330

McDonald's

Egg McMuffin 300
Large Non-fat Iced Latte w/Sugar-free Vanilla Syrup 60
Total Calories 360

Sausage Burrito 300
Small Non-fat Iced Latte 50
Total Calories 350

Fruit & Maple Oatmeal w/Brown Sugar 290
Medium Non-fat Iced Latte 60
Total Calories 350

Fruit & Maple Oatmeal w/o Brown Sugar 260
Small Non-fat Latte 90
Total Calories 350
Apple Cinnamon Walnut Oatmeal 270
Small Non-fat Iced Latte 50
Total Calories 320

Fruit & Yogurt Parfait with Granola 150
Medium Iced Latte 100
Total Calories 250

Snack Size Fruit & Walnuts with Dip 210
Small Non-fat Latte w/Sugar-free Vanilla Syrup 80
Total Calories 290

Sonic

Jr. Breakfast Burrito 260
Espresso Shot 5
Total Calories 265

Starbucks

The calorie content in Starbucks drinks certainly runs the gamut, because there are numerous options. If you do not find your favorite drink listed, then please take the time to look it up on the Starbucks website.

Spinach & Feta Egg White Wrap 280
Tall Skinny Vanilla Latte 100
Total Calories 380

Petite Vanilla Bean Scone 140
Tall Non-fat Latte w/flavored syrup 150
Total Calories 290

Perfect Oatmeal w/Brown Sugar 150
Tall Non-fat Caramel Macchiato 140
Total Calories 290

Marshmallow Dream Bar 210
Grande Iced Skinny Latte w/sugar-free syrup 80
Total Calories 290

Perfect Oatmeal with dried fruit, nut medley, & brown sugar 390
Espresso 0
Total Calories 390

Reduced-fat Turkey Bacon, Egg White, Cheddar Sandwich 320
Tall Skinny Iced Latte w/Sugar-free syrup 60
Total Calories 380

Fruit cup 90
Tall Non-fat flavored Latte 150
Total Calories 240

Banana 90
Tall Non-fat Cafe Mocha 170
Total Calories 260

Greek Yogurt & Honey Parfait 290
Grande Skinny Iced Latte w/Sugar-free syrup 80
Total Calories 370

Dark Cherry Yogurt Parfait 310
Tall Skinny Iced Mocha 70
Total Calories 380

Strawberry Blueberry Yogurt Parfait 300
Tall Skinny Iced Latte w/Sugar-free syrup 60
Total Calories 360

Vanilla Almond Biscotti 150
Tall Skinny Vanilla Latte 100
Total Calories 250

Double Chocolate Biscotti 150
Tall Skinny Mocha 110
Total Calories 260

Caramel Macchiato Biscotti 170
Tall Non-fat Caramel Macchiato 140
Total Calories 310

Breakfast Sit-Down Dining

Bob Evans

Bob Evans has a "Fit From the Farm Menu" which I have noted within the list. There are also a few items from the regular menu that are low-calorie as well. I would recommend pairing your breakfast with one of the following beverages unless you order a smoothie.

Coffee with 2 Non-dairy Creamers 38
Coffee with 2 Half & Half 80
Original Cappuccino 107
Regular Size 2% Milk 105
Regular Size Apple Juice 72
Regular Size Orange Juice 85
Hot English Breakfast Tea 1
Earl Grey Tea 1
Green Tea 1
Peppermint Tea 1
Vanilla Chai Tea 0
Iced Tea, unsweetened 0
Fit From the Farm Menu
BE Fit Breakfast 352
Blueberry Banana French Toast 347
Fresh Fruit Plate with Low Fat Strawberry Yogurt 353
Fresh Fruit Dish 58
Veggie Omelet with Fresh Fruit Dish & Wheat Toast w/Jelly 311

Low-Fat Strawberry Yogurt 93

Breakfast Menu

Turkey Sausage Breakfast 340
Border Scramble Omelet with Egg Whites 402
Farmer's Market Omelet with Egg Whites 307
Garden Harvest Omelet with Egg Whites 235
Ham & Cheddar Omelet with Egg Whites 258
Sausage & Cheddar Omelet with Egg Whites 288
Western Omelet with Egg Whites 268
Blueberry Banana Mini Fruit & Yogurt Parfait 177

A la carte

You can combine the following items from the menu to create your own low-calorie meal.

1 Hard Cooked Egg 57
2 Scrambled Bob Evans Egg Lights 57
2 Scrambled Egg Whites 50
1 Slice French Toast (no topping) 163
1 cup Oatmeal, plain 91
1 Bowl Oatmeal, plain 168
1 Slice Bacon 36
1 Turkey Sausage Link 72

Smoothies

Strawberry Banana Smoothie 256
Strawberry Blueberry Smoothie 233
Strawberry Smoothie 263

IHOP

IHOP offers several SIMPLE & FIT menu options. Some of them are still a bit of a calorie splurge. Save the calorie splurges for Saturday or Sunday brunch. IHOP does not have as many low-calorie drink options as Bob Evan's so make sure to account for those added calories when you choose your breakfast order. If you splurge on an iced mocha, then consider ordering a SIMPLE & FIT fruit bowl (130 calories) or something light a la carte.

Beverages
Coffee 5
Iced Coffee, Original 150
Iced Coffee, Mocha 200
Iced Coffee, Vanilla 190
Flavored Coffee, French Vanilla 190
Flavored Coffee, Swiss Mocha 220
Apple Juice, 10 oz. 120
Cranberry Juice, 10 oz. 130
Grapefruit Juice, 10 oz. 120
Premium Orange Juice, 10 oz. 110
Tomato Juice, 10 oz. 50
2% Milk, 10 oz. 120
Chocolate Milk, 10 oz. 220
Iced Tea, 16 oz. 10
Hot Tea 5
Herbal Tea 0
Bottled Water 0

SIMPLE & FIT

Spinach, Mushroom, Tomato Omelet 330
Turkey Bacon Omelet 420
Veggie Omelet 320
Two-Egg Breakfast 350
Oatmeal 290
Whole Wheat French Toast Combo 490
Seasonal Fresh Fruit Crepes 580
Fresh Fruit & Yogurt Bowl 330
Fruit Bowl 130
Senior Buttermilk Pancakes (3) 490

55+ Specialty Entrees

Senior Omelet, Plain w/Egg Substitute 420
Add American, Provolone, or Swiss Cheese 160
Add Bacon 80
Add Diced Ham 30
Add Green Peppers & Onions 10
Add Tomatoes 10
Add Fresh Spinach 15
Add Mushrooms 10
Senior Buttermilk Pancakes (3) 490
Senior Rooty 370
Add Compote w/Whipped Topping 90-100

Syrups per 1 oz. Serving (Use sparingly.)

Sugar-free Syrup 15
Blueberry Syrup 110
Boysenberry Syrup 100
Butter Pecan Syrup 110
Regular Old Fashioned Maple Syrup 110
Strawberry Syrup 100

Breakfast At Home

Just as a reminder, you may substitute in another beverage besides the one I have listed in the following meals if you watch the calories. Here are some possible substitutions:

Beverages

Unsweetened Green Tea 0 (Top Pick!)
Coffee with 2 Tbsp. Half & Half 40
Coffee with 1 Tbsp. Non-Dairy Flavored Creamer 35
Coffee with 2 Tbsp. Non-Dairy Flavored Creamer 70
8 oz. Skim Milk 90
8 oz. 1% Milk 105
8 oz. 2% Milk 122
4.5 oz. Chocolate Skim Milk 90
8 oz. Original Soy Milk Light 60
8 oz. Vanilla Soy Milk Light 70
8 oz. Chocolate Soy Milk Light 90
8 oz. Original Pure Coconut Milk 80
8 oz. Original Almond Milk 60
8 oz. Unsweetened Vanilla Almond Milk 40
8 oz. Vanilla Almond Milk 90
8 oz. Chocolate Almond Milk 90
8 oz. Orange Juice Light 50
4 oz. Orange Juice 55
8 oz. POM Pomegranate Juice Light 75
8 oz. Big Train Fit Frappe Protein Drink, prepared (Assorted Flavors) 60 - 70

8.25 oz. Muscle Milk Light (Assorted Flavors, Lactose Free) 100
11 oz. EAS AdvantEdge Carb Control Shake (Assorted Flavors) 110

Oatmeal

To prepare the oatmeal in this section you may follow the instructions on the package. However, I prefer my oatmeal to be the consistency of cookie batter especially with the flavor combinations that I have suggested. I add ¼ cup of boiling water per packet. I buy the oatmeal packets for convenience. If you are buying the oatmeal by the container, then just measure a heaping 1/3 cup (1/3 cup is 93 calories).

Fast & Easy Oatmeal & Egg
Plain Instant Oatmeal Packet 100
1 Hard-boiled egg 70
11 oz. EAS AdvantEdge Carb Control Shake 110
Total Calories 280

Wild Blueberry Oatmeal
Plain Instant Oatmeal Packet 100
1 cup Frozen Wild Blueberries (thawed) 70
11 oz. EAS AdvantEdge Carb Control Shake 110
Total Calories 280

Chocolate Hazelnut Oatmeal
Plain Instant Oatmeal Packet 100

1 Tbsp. Nutella 100
8.25 oz. Muscle Milk Light 100
Total Calories 300

Chocolate Banana Oatmeal
Plain Instant Oatmeal Packet 100
1 tsp. Nutella 33
1 Small Banana 90
8 oz. Original Almond Milk 60
Total Calories 283

PB & Banana Oatmeal
Plain Instant Oatmeal Packet 100
1 tsp. Natural Peanut Butter 32
1 Small Banana 90
8 oz. Original Almond Milk 60
Total Calories 282

PB & J Oatmeal
Plain Instant Oatmeal Packet 100
2 tsp. Natural Peanut Butter 63
2 tsp. Bonne Maman Brand Preserves 33
8 oz. Original Almond Milk 60
Total Calories 260

PB Chocolate Chip Oatmeal
Plain Instant Oatmeal Packet 100
2 tsp. Natural Peanut Butter 63
1 Tbsp. Semi-sweet Chocolate Chips 70
8 oz. Original Almond Milk 60
Total Calories 293

Cherry Pecan Oatmeal
Plain Instant Oatmeal Packet 100
1 Tbsp. Bonne Maman Brand Cherry Preserves 50
5 Candied Pecans, chopped 45
8 oz. Original Almond Milk 60
Total Calories 255

Peach Cobbler Oatmeal
Plain Instant Oatmeal Packet 100
1 Tbsp. Bonne Maman Brand Peach Preserves 50
1 tsp. Brown Sugar 17
1/8th tsp. Cinnamon or Pumpkin Pie Spice 1
8 oz. Original Almond Milk 60
Total Calories 228

Pumpkin Pie Spiced Oatmeal
Plain Instant Oatmeal Packet 100
1 Tbsp. Pumpkin Puree 6
1/8th tsp. (or to taste) Pumpkin Pie Spice 1
1 Tbsp. White Chocolate Chips 70
8 oz. Original Almond Milk 60
Total Calories 237

Chocolate Chip Oatmeal
Plain Instant Oatmeal Packet 100
1 Tbsp. Semi-sweet Chocolate Chips 70
1 tsp. Brown Sugar 17
8 oz. Original Almond Milk 60
Total Calories 247

Maple Pecan Oatmeal
Plain Instant Oatmeal Packet 100
2 tsp. Maple Syrup 35
2 tsp. Brown Sugar 35
5 Candied Pecans, chopped 45
8 oz. Original Almond Milk 60
Total Calories 275

Banana Nut Oatmeal
Plain Instant Oatmeal Packet 100
1 Small Banana 90
2 tsp. Brown Sugar 35
5 Candied Pecans or Walnuts, chopped 45
8 oz. Original Almond Milk 60
Total Calories 330

White Chocolate Macadamia Nut Oatmeal
Plain Instant Oatmeal Packet 100
1/2 Tbsp. White Chocolate Chips 35
1 tsp. Brown Sugar 17
4 Macadamia Nuts, chopped 70
8 oz. Original Almond Milk 60
Total Calories 282

Double Chocolate Espresso Oatmeal
Plain Instant Oatmeal Packet 100
1 Tbsp. Semi-sweet Chocolate Chips 70
1 Tbsp. Fit Frappe Mocha Protein Powder 20
1 tsp. Instant Espresso Powder 0
8 oz. Original Almond Milk 60
Total Calories 250

Almond Mocha Protein-Packed Oatmeal
Plain Instant Oatmeal Packet 100
1 Tbsp. Fit Frappe Mocha Protein Powder 20
1 Tbsp. Semi-sweet Chocolate Chips 70
1 Tbsp. Slivered Almonds 50
8 oz. Original Almond Milk
Total Calories 300

Waffles

Waffle with Maple Syrup
1 Multi-grain or Gluten-free Waffle 100
1 Tbsp. Maple Syrup 60
8 oz. Original Almond Milk 60
Total Calories 220

Waffles & Strawberries
2 Multi-grain or Gluten-free Waffles 200
½ cup Frozen Strawberries (heated) 50
1 tsp. Maple Syrup 17
Hot Tea 0
Total Calories 267

Waffles & Blueberries
2 Multi-grain or Gluten-free Waffles 200
½ cup Frozen Blueberries 35
1 tsp. Maple Syrup 17
Hot Tea 0
Total Calories 252

Cereal

I have planned the breakfast cereal portions small to give you leeway to pair it with a higher protein source like a hard-boiled egg or poached egg (70-90 calories) or a protein shake (60-100 calories). If you add one of these sources of protein to the meal, then it will help balance out the glycemic load of the meal so that you feel full longer.

1/4 cup Grape Nuts Cereal 100
1 Hard-boiled Egg 70
8 oz. Original Almond Milk 60
Total Calories 230

1/4 cup Grape Nuts Cereal 100
8 oz. Original Almond Milk 60
25 Organic Blueberries, Fresh 20
1 Hard-boiled Egg 70
Total Calories 250

1/2 cup Fiber One Original Cereal 60
1 Hard-boiled Egg 70
8 oz. Original Almond Milk 60
8 oz. Light Orange Juice 50
Total Calories 240

1 cup Fiber One Honey Clusters 160
1 Hard-boiled Egg 70
8 oz. Original Almond Milk 60
Total Calories 290

1/2 cup Fiber One Caramel Delight 90
4 oz. Skim Milk 45
8 oz. Fit Frappe Protein Shake, prepared w/water
60
Total Calories 195

1/2 cup Fiber One Raisin Bran Clusters 85
8 oz. Original Almond Milk 60
8 oz. Light Orange Juice 50
Total Calories 195

1/2 cup Kashi GoLean Crunch Original Cereal 95
8 oz. Original Almond Milk 60
8 oz. Light Orange Juice 50
Total Calories 205

1/2 cup Kashi GoLean Crunch, Honey Almond Flax
100
8 oz. Original Almond Milk 60
8 oz. Light Orange Juice 50
Total Calories 210

1 cup Kix Cereal 88
8 oz. 1% Milk 105
Total Calories 193

1 cup Multi-grain Cheerios 110
8 oz. 1% Milk 105
Total Calories 215

Eggs

In this section I have made the assumption that you already know how to cook scrambled eggs and make French toast. However, I will explain one of the easiest, fastest, low-calorie ways to cook an egg.

Easy Microwave Poached Eggs
I have to thank my husband, Carl, for this idea. He taught me how to make perfectly poached eggs in the microwave, and it has been life-saver when I am in a hurry to get out the door in the morning. All you do is fill a small ramekin or custard dish with ¼ cup of water. Add the egg. Microwave it on high for 45 to 50 seconds. Microwave times may vary. Let the egg set for a minute until the egg white looks done. The water will be hot. When it's ready spoon the egg out with a slotted spoon, and strain it on a paper towel. One large egg is only 70 calories.

Egg & Cheese Muffin
1 Light English Muffin 100
1 Large Egg, Poached 70
1 Slice American Cheese 80
Hot Chai Tea 0
Total Calories 250

Egg White French Toast
3 Tbsp. 100% Liquid Egg Whites 25
2 slices 45-calorie Bread, 100% Multi-grain 90
Cook in frying pan w/Cooking Spray 0
1 Tbsp. Honey or 1 Tbsp. Maple Syrup 60
1 tsp. Powdered Sugar and Cinnamon 10
8 oz. Original Almond Milk 60
Total Calories 245

Scrambled Eggs w/Cheese
1 Egg, Scrambled 90
Cooking Spray 0
1 Slice American Cheese 80
Coffee 2
2 Tbsp. Non Dairy Flavored Creamer, Liquid 70
Total Calories 242

Bacon & Eggs
2 Eggs, Scrambled 180
½ tsp. Butter w/Olive Oil Spread 15
2 Slices, Center Cut Bacon 50
8 oz. Orange Juice Light 50
Total Calories 295

Egg Whites Florentine
½ cup 100% Liquid Egg Whites, scrambled 50
Cooking Spray 0
1 Slice Thin Swiss Cheese 60
Baby Spinach, wilted 7
8 oz. Original Almond Milk 60
Total Calories 177

Egg Whites Verde

½ cup 100% Liquid Egg Whites, scrambled 50
Cooking Spray 0
1 oz. Colby Jack Shredded Cheese 100
1 Tbsp. Salsa Verde (Herdez brand) 5
8 oz. Orange Juice Light 50
Total Calories 205

Bagels

Bacon, Egg, & Cheese Sandwich

4 Tbsp. 100% Liquid Egg Whites 33
1 Bagel Thin or Light English Muffin 100
1 Slice Center Cut Bacon 25
1 Slice American Cheese 80
Coffee 2
Total Calories 240

Bagel with Schmear

1 Bagel Thin 100
2 Tbsp. Whipped Cream Cheese 70
8 oz. 1% Milk 105
Total Calories 275

Lunches

For lunch I have come up with several options ranging from approximately 300 to 500 calories. There are a few splurges that go over 500 calories. It is by no means an exhaustive list of all the possible options, so feel free to make substitutions based on your own personal preferences. I recommend drinking water or unsweetened iced tea with your meal so that you are not adding any empty calories. Skip the soda, and focus on hydrating.

Lunches Fast Food

Arby's

The key at Arby's is to skip all the high-calorie sides. Pair a low-calorie sandwich with sliced apples and yogurt dip (80 calories) or a chopped side salad with light Italian dressing (100 calories). If you must have your fries, then order the value size with a junior sandwich.

Roast Beef Classic 350
Horsey Sauce 50
Apple Slices 30
Yogurt Dip 50
Total Calories 480

Roast Beef Classic 350
Arby's Sauce 15
Chopped Side Salad 80
Light Italian Dressing 20
Total Calories 465

Roast Beef Mid 440
Arby's Sauce 15
Total Calories 465

Beef 'n Cheddar Classic 440
Apple Slices 30
Total Calories 470

Deluxe Bacon Cheddar 420
Apple Slices 30
Total Calories 450

French Dip & Swiss/Au Jus 430
Apple Slices 30
Total Calories 460

Cravin' Roast Chicken 380
Chopped Side Salad 80
Light Italian Dressing 20
Total Calories 480

Chicken Tenders (3) 350
Buffalo Dipping Sauce 10
Chopped Side Salad 80
Light Italian Dressing 20
Total Calories 460

Chicken Tenders (3) 350
BBQ Dipping Sauce 50
Total Calories 400

Jr. Roast Beef 210
Value Curly or Homestyle Fries 240
Total Calories 450

Jr. Ham & Cheddar Melt 210
Value Curly or Homestyle Fries 240
Total Calories 450

Jr. Chicken Sandwich 320

Chopped Farmhouse Roast Chicken Salad 250
Balsamic Vinaigrette Dressing 130
Total Calories 380

Chopped Farmhouse Crispy Chicken Salad 430
Light Italian Dressing 20
Total Calories 450

The following sandwich options are offered regionally and may be substituted for another comparable sandwich:
Arby's Melt 330
Ham & Swiss Melt 300
Jr. Deluxe Sandwich 260

Burger King

Whopper Jr. Sandwich w/o Mayo 260
Value Size Onion Rings 150
Ketchup (1 packet) 10
Total Calories 420

Whopper Jr. Sandwich 340
Apple Slices 30
Total Calories 370

Whopper Jr. Sandwich w/ Cheese w/o Mayo 300
Value Size Onion Rings 150
Ketchup (1 packet) 10
Total Calories 460

Whopper Jr. Sandwich w/Cheese 380
Apple Slices 30
Total Calories 410

Hamburger 260
Value Size French Fries 240
Ketchup (1 packet) 10
Total Calories 510

Cheeseburger 300
Value Size Onion Rings 150
Ketchup (1 packet) 10
Total Calories 460

Double Hamburger 360
Apple Slices 30
Total Calories 390

Double Cheeseburger 440

Bacon Cheeseburger 330
Apple Slices 30
Total Calories 360

Tendergrill Chicken Sandwich 470

Tendergrill Chicken Sandwich w/o Mayo 360
Apple Slices 30
Total Calories 390

Original Chicken Sandwich w/o Mayo 420
Chicken Crisp Sandwich- Classic 470

Chicken Crisp Sandwich – Spicy 460

2 piece Homestyle Chicken Strips 240
Value Size Onion Rings 150
Ketchup (1 packet) 10
Total Calories 400

3 piece Homestyle Chicken Strips 360
Apple Slices 30
Total Calories 390

4 piece Chicken Tenders 190
Ranch Dipping Sauce (1 oz.) 140
Apple Slices 30
Total Calories 360

6 piece Chicken Tenders 290
Barbecue Dipping Sauce (1 oz.) 50
Apple Slices 30
Total Calories 370

BK Big Fish Sandwich w/o Tartar Sauce 410

BK Veggie Burger 410

BK Veggie Burger w/Cheese 450

BK Veggie Burger w/o Mayo 320
Apple Slices 30
Total Calories 350

Chicken Caesar Salad w/Tendergrill and Dressing 490

Chicken BLT Salad w/Tendergrill and Dressing 510

Chicken Apple & Cranberry Salad w/Tendergrill and Dressing 520

Ranch Crispy Chicken Wrap 370
Apple Slices 30
Total Calories 400

Honey Mustard Crispy Chicken Wrap 390

Chick-fil-A

Grilled Market Salad 200
Harvest Nut Granola 60
Berry Balsamic Vinaigrette 110
Total Calories 470

Cobb Salad 430
Hold the Charred Tomato Crispy Red Bell Peppers
Fat Free Honey Mustard Dressing 100
Total Calories 530

Asian Salad 330
Hold the Honey Thai Almonds
Hold the Garlic & Ginger Wontons
Honey Sesame Dressing 170
Total Calories 500

Grilled Chicken Club Sandwich 410
BBQ or Honey Mustard Sauce 45
Total Calories 455

Grilled Chicken Sandwich 300
BBQ or Honey Mustard Sauce 45
Side Salad 80

Light Italian Dressing 25
Total Calories 450

Chicken Sandwich (no sauce) 430
Medium Fruit cup 50
Total Calories 480

Chicken Sandwich Deluxe (no sauce) 490

Spicy Chicken Sandwich (no sauce) 490

Grilled Chicken Cool Wrap (no dressing) 340
Light Italian Dressing 25
Medium Fruit cup 50
Total Calories 415

Small Hearty Breast of Chicken Soup 140
Small Carrot & Raisin Salad 260
Total Calories 400

Large Hearty Breast of Chicken Soup 220
Side Salad 80
Buttermilk Ranch Dressing 160
Total Calories 460

Chipotle

Burritos

Burrito Tortilla (no rice or beans) 290
Barbacoa 4 oz. 170
Green Tomatillo Salsa 2 oz. 15
Cheese 1 oz. 100
Total Calories 575

Burrito Tortilla (no rice or beans) 290
Chicken 4 oz. 190
Green Tomatillo Salsa 2 oz. 15
Cheese 1 oz. 100
Total Calories 595

Burrito Tortilla (no rice or beans) 290
Carnitas 4 oz. 190
Green Tomatillo Salsa 2 oz. 15
Cheese 1 oz. 100
Total Calories 595

Burrito Tortilla (no rice or beans) 290
Steak 4 oz. 190
Green Tomatillo Salsa 2 oz. 15
Cheese 1 oz. 100
Total Calories 595

Burrito Tortilla (vegetarian, no rice) 290
Black Beans 4 oz. 120
Fajita Vegetables 2.5 oz. 20
Tomato Salsa 3.5 oz. 20
Cheese 1 oz. 100
Total Calories 550

Burrito Tortilla (vegetarian, no rice) 290
Pinto Beans 4 oz. 120
Fajita Vegetables 2.5 oz. 20
Tomato Salsa 3.5 oz. 20
Cheese 1 oz. 100
Total Calories 550

Burrito Tortilla (vegetarian, no beans) 290
Cilantro-Lime Rice 3 oz. 130
Fajita Vegetables 2.5 oz. 20
Tomato Salsa 3.5 oz. 20
Cheese 1 oz. 100
Total Calories 560

Burrito Bowls

Barbacoa Bowl (no beans) 170
Cilantro-Lime Rice 3 oz. 130
Green Tomatillo Salsa 2 oz. 15
Cheese 1 oz. 100
Sour Cream 120
Total Calories 535

Barbacoa Bowl (no rice) 170
Black Beans or Pinto Beans 120
Tomato Salsa 3.5 oz. 20
Cheese 1 oz. 100
Sour Cream 120
Total Calories 530

Chicken Bowl (no beans) 190
Cilantro-Lime Rice 3 oz. 130
Green Tomatillo Salsa 2 oz. 15
Cheese 1 oz. 100
Sour Cream 120
Total Calories 555

Chicken bowl (no rice) 190
Black Beans or Pinto Beans 120
Tomato Salsa 3.5 oz. 20
Cheese 1 oz. 100
Sour Cream 120
Total Calories 550

Carnitas Bowl (no beans) 190
Cilantro-Lime Rice 3 oz. 130
Green Tomatillo Salsa 2 oz. 15
Cheese 1 oz. 100
Sour Cream 120
Total Calories 555

Carnitas Bowl (no rice) 190
Black Beans or Pinto Beans 120
Tomato Salsa 3.5 oz. 20
Cheese 1 oz. 100
Sour Cream 120
Total Calories 550

Steak Bowl (no beans) 190
Cilantro-Lime Rice 3 oz. 130
Green Tomatillo Salsa 2 oz. 15
Cheese 1 oz. 100
Sour Cream 120
Total Calories 555

Steak Bowl (no rice) 190
Black Beans or Pinto Beans 120
Tomato Salsa 3.5 oz. 20
Cheese 1 oz. 100
Sour Cream 120
Total Calories 550

Vegetarian Bowl
Black Beans 120
Cilantro-Lime Rice 3 oz. 130
Fajita Vegetables 2.5 oz. 20
Tomato Salsa 3.5 oz. 20
Cheese 1 oz. 100
Sour Cream 120
Total Calories 510

Vegetarian Bowl (no cheese or sour cream)
Black Beans 120
Cilantro-Lime Rice 3 oz. 130
Fajita Vegetables 2.5 oz. 20
Tomato Salsa 3.5 oz. 20
Corn Salsa 3.5 oz. 80
Guacamole 3.5 oz. 150
Total Calories 520

Vegetarian Bowl (no rice)
Black Beans 120
Fajita Vegetables 2.5 oz. 20
Tomato Salsa 3.5 oz. 20
Corn Salsa 3.5 oz. 80
Cheese 1 oz. 100
Sour Cream 120
Total Calories 460

Vegetarian Bowl (no beans)
Cilantro-Lime Rice 3 oz. 130
Fajita Vegetables 2.5 oz. 20
Tomato Salsa 3.5 oz. 20
Guacamole 3.5 oz. 150
Cheese 1 oz. 100
Total Calories 420

Tacos

3 Crispy Tacos 180
Barbacoa 4 oz. 170
Green Tomatillo Salsa 2 oz. 15
Cheese 1 oz. 100
Romaine Lettuce 1 oz. 5
Total Calories 470

3 Crispy Tacos 180
Chicken 4 oz. 190
Green Tomatillo Salsa 2 oz. 15
Cheese 1 oz. 100
Romaine Lettuce 1 oz. 5
Total Calories 490

3 Crispy Tacos 180
Carnitas 4 oz. 190
Green Tomatillo Salsa 2 oz. 15
Cheese 1 oz. 100
Romaine Lettuce 1 oz. 5
Total Calories 490

3 Crispy Tacos 180
Steak 4 oz. 190
Green Tomatillo Salsa 2 oz. 15
Cheese 1 oz. 100
Romaine Lettuce 1 oz. 5
Total Calories 490

3 Crispy Tacos (vegetarian, no rice) 180
Black Beans or Pinto Beans 120
Fajita Vegetables 2.5 oz. 20
Tomato Salsa 3.5 oz. 20
Guacamole 3.5 oz. 150
Total Calories 490

3 Crispy Tacos (vegetarian, no beans) 180
Cilantro-Lime Rice 3 oz. 130
Fajita Vegetables 2.5 oz. 20
Tomato Salsa 3.5 oz. 20
Guacamole 3.5 oz. 150
Total Calories 500

Salads

Salad (no dressing) 10
Barbacoa 170
Black Beans or Pinto Beans 120
Tomato Salsa 3.5 oz. 20
Cheese 1 oz. 100
Sour Cream 120
Total Calories 540

Salad (no dressing) 10
Chicken 190
Black Beans or Pinto Beans 120
Tomato Salsa 3.5 oz. 20
Cheese 1 oz. 100
Sour Cream 120
Total Calories 560

Salad (no dressing) 10
Carnitas 190
Black Beans or Pinto Beans 120
Tomato Salsa 3.5 oz. 20
Cheese 1 oz. 100
Sour Cream 120
Total Calories 560

Salad (no dressing) 10
Steak 190
Black Beans or Pinto Beans 120
Tomato Salsa 3.5 oz. 20
Cheese 1 oz. 100
Sour Cream 120
Total Calories 560

Salad (no dressing) 10
Fajita Vegetables 2.5 oz. 20
Black Beans or Pinto Beans 120
Tomato Salsa 3.5 oz. 20
Corn Salsa 3.5 oz. 80
Cheese 1 oz. 100
Sour Cream 120
Total Calories 470

Einstein Brothers

Half Chicken Chipotle Salad 360
Chile Lime Dressing 60
Total Calories 420

Tuna Thin 250
11 Sun Chips 140
Total Calories 390

Turkey Thin 250
Italian Wedding Soup 160
Total Calories 410

Turkey-Bacon Avocado Thin 380
Total Calories 380

Pepperoni Pizza Bagel 450

Cheese Pizza Bagel 400

Spinach Florentine Bagel 340
Cream Cheese 60
Total Calories 400

Asiago Bagel 310
Cream Cheese 60
Total Calories 370

Broccoli Cheese Soup 290

Jimmy John's

8" Ham & Cheese Slim 508

Ham & Cheese Slim on Wheat Bread 509

8" Roast Beef Slim 424

Roast Beef Slim on Wheat Bread 425

8" Turkey Slim 401

Turkey Slim on Wheat Bread 402

6 Vegetarian Unwich (Lettuce Wrap) 336

#1 Pepe Unwich (Lettuce Wrap) 375

2 Big John Unwich (Lettuce Wrap) 291

3 Totally Tuna Unwich (Lettuce Wrap) 449

4 Turkey Tom Unwich (Lettuce Wrap) 272

5 Vito Unwich (Lettuce Wrap) 358

KFC

3 Crispy Chicken Strips 390

2 Crispy Chicken Strips 260
Mashed Potatoes with Gravy 120
Total Calories 380

Original Recipe Bites (6) 200
Macaroni and Cheese 160
Honey BBQ Dipping Sauce cup 40
Total Calories 400

Crispy Chicken BLT Salad 360
Ranch Fat Free Dressing 35
Total Calories 395

Original Filet 200
3" Corn on the Cob 70
Cole Slaw 180
Total Calories 450

Grilled Chicken Breast 220
Mashed Potatoes with Gravy 120
Green Beans 25
Total Calories 365

Original Chicken Breast 360
Mashed Potatoes with Gravy 120
Total Calories 480

Original Chicken Breast without skin or breading 160
Mashed Potatoes with Gravy 120
Green Beans 25
Total Calories 305

Grilled Chicken Breast 220
Grilled Chicken Whole Wing 80
3" Corn Cobbett 70
Total Calories 370

Grilled Chicken Drumstick 90
Grilled Chicken Thigh 170
Mashed Potatoes with Gravy 120
Total Calories 380

Original Chicken Drumstick 120
Original Chicken Thigh 250
Green Beans 25
Total Calories 395

Extra Crispy Chicken Drumstick 150
Mashed Potatoes with Gravy 120
Cole Slaw 180
Total Calories 450

Spicy Crispy Drumstick 160
Mashed Potatoes with Gravy 120
Total Calories 280

Long John Silver's

Baked Cod Meal (no hushpuppies)
Baked Cod 1 piece 160
Seasoned Green Beans 29
Corn Cobbette without Butter Oil 90
Rice 180
Total Calories 459

Baked Shrimp Meal
8 Baked Shrimp 67
Seasoned Green Beans 29
Corn Cobbette without Butter Oil 90
Rice 180
2 Hushpuppies 160
Total Calories 526

Cranberry Walnut Chicken Salad 390
Raspberry Vinaigrette 45
Total Calories 435

Ciabata Jack Fish Sandwich 550

1 Baja Fish Taco 580

1 Baja Chicken Taco 530

1 Battered Alaskan Pollock 230
Corn Cobbette without Butter Oil 90
Seasoned Green Beans 29
Total Calories 349

1 Battered Cod 280
1 Tartar Sauce packet 40
Seasoned Green Beans 29
Total Calories 349

3 Battered Shrimp 130
1 Battered Cod 280
Cocktail Sauce (1 dipping cup) 25
Total Calories 435

Popcorn Shrimp 330
Cocktail Sauce (1 dipping cup) 25
Total Calories 355

1 Chicken Tender 170
Cole Slaw 200
Total Calories 370

2 Chicken Tenders 340
Seasoned Green Beans 29
Total Calories 369

Buttered Langostino Lobster Bites 230
Corn Cobbette without Butter Oil 90
Total Calories 320

Crab Cake 280
3 Battered Shrimp 130
Cocktail Sauce (1 dipping cup) 25
Seasoned Green Beans 29
Total Calories 464

McDonald's

Hamburger 250
Small Fries 230
Total Calories 480

Cheeseburger 300
Small Fries 230
Total Calories 530

Quarter Pounder with Cheese 520

Double Cheeseburger 440

Filet O' Fish 380
Apple Slices 15
Total Calories 395

Premium Grilled Chicken Classic 350
Apple Slices 15
Total Calories 365

Premium Grilled Chicken Club 460
Apple Slices 15
Total Calories 475

Premium Grilled Chicken Ranch BLT 380
Apple Slices 15
Total Calories 395

McChicken 360
Apple Slices 15
Total Calories 375

Honey Mustard or Chipotle BBQ Snack Wrap
(grilled) 250
Small French Fries 230
Total Calories 490

Angus Bacon & Cheese Snack Wrap 390
Apple Slices 15
Total Calories 405

Angus Deluxe Snack Wrap 410
Side Salad 20
Low Fat Balsamic Dressing 35
Total Calories 465

Honey Mustard or Chipotle BBQ Snack Wrap
(crispy) 330
Fruit & Yogurt Parfait with Granola 150
Total Calories 480

Ranch Wrap (crispy) 350
Fruit & Yogurt Parfait with Granola 150
Total Calories 500

Ranch Wrap (grilled) 270
Fruit & Yogurt Parfait with Granola 150
Total Calories 420

Side Salad 20
Low Fat Balsamic Dressing 35
Snack Size Fruit & Walnuts 210
Total Calories 265

Premium Bacon Ranch Salad 140
Creamy Southwest Dressing 100
Snack Size Fruit & Walnuts 210
Total Calories 440

Premium Bacon Ranch Salad w/Grilled Chicken 230
Low Fat Balsamic Dressing 35
Fruit & Yogurt Parfait with Granola 150
Total Calories 415

Premium Bacon Ranch Salad w/Grilled Chicken 230
Ranch Dressing 170
Total Calories 400

Premium Caesar Salad 90
Caesar Dressing 190
Butter Garlic Croutons 60
Total Calories 340

Premium Caesar Salad w/Grilled Chicken 190
Caesar Dressing 190
Butter Garlic Croutons 60
Total Calories 440

Premium Southwest Salad 140
Creamy Southwest Dressing 100
Total Calories 240

Premium Southwest Salad w/Grilled Chicken 290
Creamy Southwest Dressing 100
Total Calories 390

Panda Express

Panda Bowl Kung Pao Shrimp w/Mixed Veggies 320

Panda Bowl Tangy Shrimp w/Mixed Veggies 260

Panda Bowl Crispy Shrimp w/Mixed Veggies 330

Panda Bowl Honey Walnut Shrimp w/Mixed Veggies 440

Panda Bowl Fried Rice w/Mixed Veggies 380

Panda Bowl Chow Mein Noodles w/Mixed Veggies 290

Panda Bowl Steamed Rice w/Mixed Veggies 290

Panda Bowl String Bean Chicken w/Mixed Veggies 240

Panda Bowl Broccoli Beef w/ Chow Mein/Mixed Veggies 440

Panda Bowl Mushroom Chicken w/Mixed Veggies 290

Panda Bowl Black Pepper Chicken w/Mixed Veggies 320

Egg Flower Soup 90
Side of Mixed Veggies 70
Veggie Spring Rolls (2) 160
Total Calories 320

Hot & Sour Soup 90
Side of Mixed Veggies 70
Crab Rangoon (3) 190
Total Calories 350

Panera

Choose from the *You Pick Two Menu*. Skip all the add-ons or grab the apple for an afternoon snack.

1/2 French Onion Soup (no Cheese/no Crouton) 80
1/2 Asiago Roast Beef 350
Total Calories 430

French Onion Soup w/ Cheese & Crouton 210
1/2 Greek Salad 190
Total Calories 400

Greek Salad 380

Baked Potato Soup 250
1/2 Classic Cafe Salad 80
Total Calories 330

Brocolli Cheddar Soup 190
1/2 Chicken Cobb Chopped Salad 250
Total Calories 440

Pizza Hut

This is a calorie splurge! Consider reserving this for dinner.

6" Personal Pan Cheese Pizza 590

6" Personal Pan Veggie Lover's Pizza 550

Popeye's

Mild Chicken Breast 440
Regular Green Beans 40
Total Calories 480

Spicy Chicken Breast 420
Cajun Rice 170
Total Calories 590

Mild Chicken Leg 160
Mild Chicken Thigh 280
Regular Green Beans 40
Total Calories 480

Spicy Chicken Leg 170
Spicy Chicken Thigh 260
Regular Green Beans 40
Total Calories 470

Regular Red Beans & Rice 230

Naked Chicken Strips (3 pieces) 170
Regular Mashed Potatoes & Gravy 120
Total Calories 290

Spicy Chicken Tenders (3 pieces) 310
Regular Mashed Potatoes & Gravy 120
Total Calories 430

Popcorn Shrimp 330
Cajun Rice 170
Total Calories 500

Butterfly Shrimp (8 shrimp) 290
Cocktail Sauce 30
Cajun Rice 170
Total Calories 490

Chicken Nuggets (6 pieces) 230
Barbecue Sauce 45
Cajun Rice 170
Total Calories 445

Chicken Sausage Jambalaya 220
Biscuit 260
Total Calories 480

Loaded Chicken Wrap 310

Chicken Biscuit 490

Sonic

Grilled Chicken Bacon Ranch 470

Small 4 oz. Jumbo Popcorn Chicken 380
BBQ Sauce 45
Total Calories 425

Grilled Chicken Wrap 390
Apple Slices (no dipping sauce) 35
Total Calories 425

Crispy Chicken Wrap 490

Grilled Chicken Salad 250
Light Ranch Dressing 70
Total Calories 320

Crispy Chicken Salad 340
Light Ranch Dressing 70
Total Calories 410

Jr. Burger 340
Apple Slices (no dipping sauce) 35
Total Calories 375

Jr. Deluxe Burger 380
Apple Slices (no dipping sauce) 35
Total Calories 415

Jr. Deluxe Cheeseburger 450
Apple Slices (no dipping sauce) 35
Total Calories 485

Veggie Burger (w/mustard or ketchup) 450
Apple Slices (no dipping sauce) 35
Total Calories 485

Grilled Cheese 410
Apple Slices (no dipping sauce) 35
Total Calories 445

BLT Toaster Sandwich 550

Chicken Strips (2) 200
Small Tater Tots 130
1 Ketchup 9
Total Calories 339

Chicken Strips (3} 300
Apple Slices (no dipping sauce) 35
Total Calories 335

Chicken Strip Sandwich 450
Apple Slices (no dipping sauce) 35
Total Calories 485

All Beef Regular Hot Dog (6") 320
Small Tots 130
1 Ketchup 9
Total Calories 459

All Beef New York Dog (6") 340
Small Tots 130
1 Ketchup 9
Total Calories 479

All Beef All-American Dog (6") 370
Apple Slices (no dipping sauce) 35
Total Calories 405

All Beef Chicago Dog (6") 430
Apple Slices (no dipping sauce) 35
Total Calories 465

All Beef Chili Cheese Coney (6"] 410
Apple Slices (no dipping sauce) 35
Total Calories 445

Corn Dog 210
Small Tots 130
1 Ketchup 9
Total Calories 349

Subway

All Subway Sandwiches listed include the veggies.

6" Veggie Delite on 9-Grain Wheat Bread 230
American Cheese (2 Triangles) 40
Light Mayo 50
Mustard 5
Dannon Light & Fit Yogurt 80
Total Calories 405

6" Sweet Onion Teriyaki on 9-Grain Wheat Bread 380
American Cheese (2 Triangles) 40
Apple Slices 35
Total Calories 455

6" Black Forest Ham on 9-Grain Wheat Bread 290
American Cheese (2 Triangles) 40
Light Mayo 50
Mustard 5
Baked Lays 130
Total Calories 515

6" Turkey Breast on 9-Grain Wheat Bread 280
American Cheese (2 Triangles) 40
Light Mayo 50
Mustard 5
Baked Lays 130
Total Calories 505

6" Roast Beef on 9-Grain Wheat Bread 310
American Cheese (2 Triangles) 40
Light Mayo 50
Mustard 5
Dannon Light & Fit Yogurt 80
Total Calories 485

6" Club on 9-Grain Wheat Bread 320
American Cheese (2 Triangles) 40
Light Mayo 50
Mustard 5
Dannon Light & Fit Yogurt 80
Total Calories 495

6" Turkey and Ham on 9-Grain Wheat Bread 300
American Cheese (2 Triangles) 40
Light Mayo 50
Mustard 5
Dannon Light & Fit Yogurt 80
Total Calories 475

6" Oven Roasted Chicken on 9-Grain Wheat Bread 320
American Cheese (2 Triangles) 40
Light Mayo 50
Mustard 5
Dannon Light & Fit Yogurt 80
Total Calories 495

Taco Bell

Beef Burrito Supreme 420

7 Layer Burrito 500

Bean Burrito 370
Fresco Ranchero Chicken Soft Taco 170
Total Calories 540

Beefy Nacho Burrito 470

Chicken Burrito Supreme 400

Steak Burrito Supreme 390

Chicken Burrito 430

Chili Cheese Burrito 380

Fresco Bean Burrito 350

Chicken Chalupa Supreme 370

Steak Chalupa Supreme 360

Beef Chalupa Supreme 390

Fresco Chicken Burrito Supreme 350

Fresco Steak Burrito Supreme 340

Fresco Chicken Soft Taco 150
Fresco Crunch Taco 150
Total Calories 300

Fresco Grilled Steak Soft Taco 150
Fresco Soft Taco 180
Total Calories 330

Cheesy Gordita Crunch 490

Chicken Gordita Supreme 270
Fresco Crunchy Taco 150
Total Calories 420

Steak Gordita Supreme 270
Fresco Chicken Soft Taco 150
Total Calories 420

Beef Gordita Supreme 300
Mexican Rice 120
Total Calories 420

Cheesy Nachos 280
Fresco Chicken Soft Taco 150
Total Calories 430

Nachos 330

Nachos Supreme 440

Pintos n' Cheese 170
Fresco Chicken Soft Taco 150
Total Calories 320

Mexican Pizza 540

Steak Quesadilla 520

Cheese Quesadilla 480

Tostada 250
Mexican Rice 120
Total Calories 370

Cheese Roll-up 190
Pintos n' Cheese 170
Total Calories 360

Crunchwrap Supreme 540

Chicken Enchirito 340

Steak Enchirito 330

Beef Enchirito 360

Express Taco Salad w/Chips 580

Chicken Soft Taco 180
Crispy Potato Soft Taco 270
Total Calories 450

Crunchy Taco 170
Crunchy Taco Supreme 200
Total Calories 370

Double Decker Taco Supreme 350

Doritos Locos Tacos Supreme 200
Grilled Steak Soft Taco 250
Total Calories 450

Double Decker Taco 320

Beef Soft Taco Supreme 230
Beef Soft Taco 200
Total Calories 430

Crunchy Taco 170
Crispy Potato Soft Taco 270
Total Calories 440

Meximelt 270
Crunchy Taco 170
Total Calories 440

Chicken Soft Taco 180
Crunchy Taco 170
Total Calories 350

Wendy's

5 piece Chicken Nuggets 230
Honey Mustard 130
Apple Slices 40
Total Calories 400

Grilled Chicken Go Wrap 260
Side Caesar Salad w/ Caesar Dressing & Croutons
250
Total Calories 510

Jr. Cheeseburger Deluxe (no bacon) 300
Garden Side Salad w/ Ancho Chipotle Ranch
Dressing & Croutons 220
Total Calories 520

Ultimate Chicken Grill Sandwich 350
Apple Slices 40
Total Calories 390

Ultimate Chicken Grill Sandwich (no bun) 180
Sour Cream & Chive Baked Potato 320
Total Calories 500

Spicy Chicken Sandwich (no bun, no mayo) 240
Garden Side Salad w/ Ranch Dressing (no croutons)
200
Total Calories 440

Full-sized Asian Cashew Chicken Salad 210
Spicy Roasted Cashews 80
Light Spicy Chili Vinaigrette Dressing 90
Total Calories 380

Half-sized BBQ Chicken Ranch Salad 160
Honey BBQ Glaze 30
Applewood Smoked Bacon 25
BBQ Ranch Dressing 100
Total Calories 310

Half-sized Apple Pecan Chicken Salad 180
Roasted Pecans 110
Pomegranate Vinaigrette Dressing 60
Total Calories 350

Half-sized Spicy Chicken Caesar Salad 240
Croutons 80
Lemon Caesar Dressing 110
Total Calories 430

Lunches At Home

The great thing about eating lunch at home is that it is easy to make healthier choices if you have the right groceries on hand. You have to plan ahead, but it is worth it. I find it so much easier to have a healthy, high-fiber, filling, low-calorie lunch at home. The portions are larger and ultimately more satisfying.

Some of the options I have listed are easy to make ahead for a packed lunch. Some require a microwave or a stove. If you do not have access to a stove at work, then save the grilled cheese for your day off.

I did not go into detailed instructions on many of the items, because I operated on the assumption that you know how make a Panini, grilled cheese, etc. For meals that are not as self-explanatory I included the recipe.

Just as I did with the fast food lunch options I tried to come up with several meal options ranging from approximately 300 to 500 calories. As a reminder I still recommend drinking water or unsweetened iced tea with your meal so that you are not adding any empty calories.

PB Sandwich & Crudité
2 slices 45-Calorie Wheat Bread 90
(I like Sara Lee or Pepperidge Farm brand.)
1 Tbsp. Skippy Natural Peanut Butter 85
1 Celery Stalk 6
5 Baby Carrots 18
1 Small Organic Apple 77
Total Calories 276

Bacon Ranch Salad
1 cup Mixed Greens 13
Hard Boiled Egg 70
1 Tbsp. Real Bacon Bits 30
1/4 cup Peas 31
1/4 cup Chickpeas 71
1/4 cup Kidney beans 52
2 Tbsp. Bolthouse Farms Yogurt Ranch Dressing 70
Total Calories 337

Wedge Salad & Summer Vegetable Soup
¼ Head of Iceberg Lettuce 19
2 Tbsp. Blue Cheese Crumbles 75
2 Tbsp. Bolthouse Farms Chunky Blue Cheese Yogurt Dressing 35
½ cup Fresh Diced Tomatoes 16
4 slices Ready to Serve Fully Cooked Bacon, crumbled 70
1 cup Amy's Organic Summer Corn & Vegetable Soup 150
Total Calories 365

Grilled Cheese & Tomato Soup

2 slices 45-Calorie Wheat Bread 90
2 slices American Cheese 160
1 Tbsp. Brummel & Brown Spread 45
1 cup Amy's Organic Cream of Tomato Soup 110
Total Calories 405

Italian Grilled Cheese & Minestrone

2 slices 45-Calorie Wheat Bread 90
1 Slice Provolone Cheese 80
1 Slice Smoked Mozzarella or Smoked Gouda 100
1 Slice Fresh Tomato 5
2 Fresh Basil Leaves, chifonade 0
1 Tbsp. Brummel & Brown Spread 45
1 cup Amy's Organic Minestrone Soup 90
Total Calories 410

Easy Gorgonzola Mushroom Soup & Cheesy Texas Toast

1 cup Gluten-Free Café Brand Cream of Mushroom Soup 90
½ oz. Gorgonzola Cheese, to garnish the soup 50
1 Slice New York Brand Five Cheese Texas Toast 180
Total Calories 320

Turkey, Brie, Fig Jam Panini & Chips

2 slices 45-Calorie Wheat Bread 90
2 oz. Deli Turkey 60
1 oz. Brie 95
1 Tbsp. Fig Jam 50
20 Kettle Chips, Baked, Sea Salt 120
Total Calories 415

Easy French Onion Soup Gratin

1 cup Wolfgang Puck French Onion Soup 80
1 Tbsp. Gruyere, shredded 40
1 Slice New York Brand Five Cheese Texas Toast 180
Bake the bread according to instructions. Lay the toast in on top of the soup in an oven-safe crock. Top with gruyere. Bake in a 350 degree until cheese is melted and soup is hot. Broil on high for 30-60 seconds until cheese is golden brown.
Total Calories 300

Philly-Style Panini & Mushroom Soup

2 Slices 45-Calorie Wheat Bread 90
2 oz. Deli Roast Beef 90
1 slice Provolone Cheese 80
1 oz. Sautéed Onions & Peppers, cooked with cooking spray 8
Cooking Spray, to cook the Panini 0
1 cup Gluten-Free Café Brand Cream of Mushroom Soup 90
Total Calories 358

Beef w/Blue Cheese Wrap & Chips
1 Flatout Flatbread Light 90
2 oz. Deli Roast Beef 90
¼ cup Baby Spinach 5
½ oz. Gorgonzola or Blue Cheese, crumbled 50
20 Kettle Chips, Baked, Sea Salt 120
Total Calories 355

Rueben & Pickle Spear
2 Slices Pumpernickel Rye Bread (Pepperidge Farm) 160
2 oz. Pastrami or Corned Beef 80
¼ cup Sauerkraut 5
1 Tbsp. Thousand Island dressing 60
1 Slice Swiss Cheese 100
1 Dill Pickle Spear 5
Total Calories 410

½ Rachel & Chips
1 Slice Marble Rye Bread, cut in half 80
2 oz. Deli Turkey or Turkey Pastrami 70
¼ cup Sauerkraut 5
2 tsp. Thousand Island dressing 40
1 Slice Swiss Cheese 100
20 Kettle Chips, Baked, Sea Salt 120
Total Calories 415

California Deli Sandwich & Chips
2 slices 45-Calorie Wheat Bread 90
4 oz. Deli Meat (Turkey or Ham) 120
1 Tbsp. Light Mayo 35
1/2 cup Mixed Greens 5
Tomato Slice 5
1/4 Avocado 72
10 Kettle Chips, Baked, Aged White Cheddar 60
Total Calories 387

Deli Sandwich & Grapes
2 slices 45-Calorie Wheat Bread 90
1/2 cup Alfalfa Sprouts or 1 cup Mixed Greens 13
2 oz. Deli Ham or Turkey 60
1 slice Provolone Cheese 80
1 Tbsp. Light Mayo 35
20 Grapes 68
Total Calories 346

Tuna Veggie Roll & Mushroom Rice Noodle Bowl

Ingredients
1 Star-Kist Single Serve Sweet & Spicy Tuna Pouch
1 Celery Stalk, cut into thin julienne strips
1/2 Cucumber, peeled, seeded, cut into thin strips
1 Tbsp. Light Mayonnaise
1/8 tsp. Wasabi Powder or Paste
1 Asian Rice Spring Roll Wrapper
1 Tbsp. Soy Sauce for dipping

Directions
Mix the wasabi powder or paste into the mayo.
Wet the rice wrapper on a plate of water. Shake off
the excess. Stack the veggies and tuna in the center
of the wrapper. Top with wasabi mayo. Roll tightly
like a burrito. You can add more wasabi to the soy
sauce for dipping.

Number of Servings: 1

Nutrition Information/Serving:

Calories: 181
Fat: 4g
Carbohydrates: 30g
Protein: 21g

Serve with:
1 Thai Kitchen Mushroom Rice Noodle Bowl 240
Total Calories 421

California Sushi Rolls
(On average for 8 small rolls from the grocer) 300
1 Tbsp. Soy Sauce 11
Unsweetened Green Tea 0
Total Calories 311

Burger & Fries
Smart Ones Mini Cheeseburger (1) 200
Ore Ida Easy Fries (22 pieces) 170
1 Tbsp. Organic ketchup 20
Total Calories 390

Frank & Beans
1 Beef Frank 149
1/2 cup Baked Beans, canned 110
1 Light Hot Dog Bun (like Sara Lee) 80
1 tsp. Dijon Mustard 5
Total Calories 344

Veggie Pita Pizza

Ingredients
1 White or Wheat Pita (6.5" diameter)
¼ cup 6-Cheese Italian Blend, shredded
1 oz. Canned Diced Tomatoes, drained
½ Tbsp. Grated Parmesan
8 Sliced Mushrooms, raw
1 oz. Marinated Artichoke Quarters, drained
6 Sweet Pepper Strips, raw
1 Tbsp. Sliced Black Olives

Directions
Spread the diced tomatoes on the pita. Top with grated parmesan and shredded cheese. Top with the vegetables. Heat in the microwave until the cheese is melted.

Serving Size: 1 pizza

Nutrition Information/Serving:

Calories: 333
Fat: 12g
Carbohydrates: 44g
Protein: 16g

Spinach & Mushroom Flatbread

Ingredients
1 Flatout Flatbread Light, toasted under broiler until crisp
1 Tbsp. Classico Roasted Garlic Alfredo Sauce
1 Tsp. Grated Parmesan
¼ cup 6-Cheese Italian Blend, shredded
½ cup Mushrooms (Shitake,Oyster,Cremini), raw
½ cup Organic Baby Spinach, fresh, chopped
1 Tbsp. Brummel & Brown Spread
1 Tsp. Minced Garlic, jarred
Fresh Grated Nutmeg, Salt & Pepper to taste
¼ tsp. Truffle Oil (optional)

Directions
Sauté the mushrooms in the Brummel & Brown spread on medium heat. Once the mushrooms look close to done add the spinach, garlic, and seasonings. Remove from the heat as soon as the spinach is wilted.

Toast the flatbread under the broiler until crisp. Make sure to keep an eye on it so it doesn't burn.

Top the flatbread with Alfredo sauce, parmesan, and cheese blend. Top with sautéed mushrooms and spinach.

Broil on low heat and watch for the cheese to bubble. Remove from the oven and drizzle with a tiny bit of truffle oil. I prefer Oilerie Truffle Oil from Oilerie.com.

Serving Size: 1 pizza

Nutrition Information/Serving:

Calories: 282
Fat: 18g
Carbohydrates: 21g
Protein: 19g

Easy Veggie Quesadilla

Ingredients
1/4 cup Birds Eye The Ultimate Southwest Blend, thawed (black beans, corn, onions, chilies)
1/4 cup 2% Milk Shredded Sharp Cheddar Cheese
1 Mission Low Carb Taco Size Flour Tortilla
2 Tbsp. Pico de Gallo
2 Tbsp. Reduced Fat Sour Cream
Cooking spray

Directions
Spray a skillet with cooking spray. Heat on Medium High Heat. Thaw and drain the southwest blend. Fill the tortilla with the vegetable blend, and cheese. Fold and heat on each side for about 5 minutes. Top with Pico de Gallo and sour cream.

Serving Size: 1 quesadilla

Nutrition Information/Serving:

Calories: 274
Fat: 13g
Carbohydrates: 28g
Protein: 16g

Bacon Avocado Egg Salad

Ingredients

4 Large Hard-Boiled Eggs, chopped (I like Eggland's Best Hard-Cooked Peeled Eggs for convenience.)
2 Slices Center Cut Bacon, Cooked and Crumbled
1/2 Ripe Avocado, cubed or mashed
1 Tbsp. Reduced Fat Olive Oil Mayo
2 Tbsp. Non-Fat Greek Yogurt
1 Tbsp. Fresh Lime Juice
Salt and Pepper to Taste
1/4 tsp. Cayenne Pepper (optional)

Directions

Mix all the ingredients in a bowl. Serve on an 80-calorie wheat bun or a bed of mixed greens.

Serving Size: 1/2 recipe

Nutrition Information/Serving:

Calories: 244
Fat: 17g
Carbohydrates: 6g
Protein: 14g

Curry Chicken Salad

Ingredients
8 oz. Cooked Chicken Breast
1/4 cup Golden Raisins
1 tsp curry powder
2 Tbsp. Light Mayonnaise
3 Tbsp. Plain Nonfat Yogurt
1/4 cup almonds, slivered
2 Tbsp. cilantro (optional)

Directions
Cut the chicken into 1-inch cubes. Mix all the ingredients together. Serve as lettuce wraps using romaine or leaf lettuce.

Number of Servings: 2

Nutrition Information/Serving:

Calories: 310
Fat: 12g
Carbohydrates: 22g
Protein: 31g

Or serve with:
 Light Wheat Bun (like Sara Lee) 80
1 oz. Leaf Lettuce 4
Total Calories 394

Buffalo Chicken Salad

Ingredients
8 oz. Cooked Chicken Breast
1 celery stalk, diced
4 Tbsp. Light Mayonnaise
2 oz. Blue Cheese or Gorgonzola, crumbled
3 tsp. Cayenne Pepper Sauce, or to taste
Salt and Pepper to taste

Directions
Chop the chicken breasts into 1-inch cubes. Mix all the ingredients in a bowl and serve immediately on low-calorie bread as a sandwich or over mixed greens as a salad.

Number of Servings: 2

Nutrition Information/Serving:

Calories: 300
Fat: 17g
Carbohydrates: 3g
Protein: 32g

Or serve with:
Light Wheat Bun (like Sara Lee) 80
1 oz. Leaf Lettuce 4
1 oz. Baby Carrots 10
Total Calories 394

Santa Fe Chicken Salad Sliders

Ingredients
12 oz. of Grilled Chicken Breasts
1/4 cup canned Black Beans, drained and rinsed
1/4 cup yellow sweet corn, thawed
1/4 cup low fat sour cream
1/2 cup of prepared Pico de Gallo (or make your own fresh tomato, onion, jalapeno, cilantro, and lime juice)
4 Romaine lettuce leaves
4 Whole Wheat Slider-size Rolls

Directions
Chop the chicken breasts into 1-inch cubes. Mix with the beans, corn, sour cream, and Pico de Gallo. Salt and pepper to taste.

Serve with romaine lettuce on whole wheat rolls. Add some veggies on the side for a well-balanced lunch.

Serving Size: 4 servings

Nutrition Information/Serving:

Calories: 225
Fat: 5g
Carbohydrates: 21g
Protein: 24g

From The Grocer's Freezer

This section reflects some of my own personal preferences. I have tried a lot of low-calorie entrees and pizzas. Some brands impress me more than others so I have purposely left certain brands/items out. If I felt like a frozen entrée was a waste of my money, then it definitely did not make the list.

I do not recommend eating a lot of over-processed food. These foods should be limited in your diet. Fresh food tends to be better in terms of taste and nutrition. Eating a lot of processed food disrupts your endocrine system and slows down your metabolism. However, we all have those moments when we get in a hurry or just do not feel like cooking an elaborate meal.

Having a freezer stocked with tasty, low-calorie options makes it really easy to stay on track. If nothing else it provides portion control. Grab an entrée when you don't have time to pack a more elaborate lunch. For an easy dinner add a lightly dressed side salad, a cup of soup, or a piece of fruit to one of these entrees to round out your meal.

Amy's Kitchen

This is my favorite brand, because it offers a lot of organic, vegetarian, and gluten-free items. I have not tried every product, but here are my favorites!

Mexican Tamale Pie 150
Black Bean Tamale Verde 330
Cheese Tamale Verde 400
Enchilada Verde 400
Roasted Vegetable Tamale 280
Macaroni & Cheese 400
Vegetable Lasagna 310
Roasted Vegetable Lasagna 350
Mexican Casserole Bowl 380
Pesto Tortellini Bowl 430
Stuffed Pasta Shells Bowl 310
Light & Lean Spinach Lasagna 250
Indian Mattar Paneer 370

California Pizza Kitchen

The small pizzas are a godsend. Here's the skinny on the calorie content of my favorites.

1 Small Margherita 390
1 Small Four Cheese 400
1 Small Hawaiian 350
1 Small BBQ Chicken 390
1 Small Sicilian 420

For the Larger Crispy Thin Crust or Original Crust frozen pizzas stick to a single serving of 1/3 of the pizza.

Lean Cuisine

Garlic Chicken Spring Rolls 200
Fajita Style Chicken Spring Rolls 200
Thai Style Chicken Spring Rolls 200
Butternut Squash Ravioli 260
Beef Portobello 200
Asian Style Pot Stickers 260
Roasted Turkey Breast 290
Glazed Turkey Tenderloins 250
Swedish Meatballs with Pasta 290
Spinach & Mushroom Deep Dish Pizza 340
Three Meat Pizza Deep Dish 390
Asiago Cheese Tortelloni 270

Smart Ones

(I often add 2 tsp. Of Grated Parmesan and fresh cracked pepper to these entrees for a little more flavor. The Parmesan adds 20 calories which is not included in the list.)

Pasta with Ricotta and Spinach 300
Mini Rigatoni with Vodka Cream Sauce 290
Pasta Primavera 250
Ravioli Florentine 270
Three Cheese Ziti Marinara 300
Lasagna Florentine 310

Snacks

There are lots of 100-calorie snack packs out there, but a lot of them aren't very satisfying. Snack packs are often full of sugar and low on fiber. I'm not saying you should not indulge in the occasional 100-calorie snack pack of sweets, however there are some other snack options that are more satiating. The key to a satisfying snack is balance. Look for high fiber options, protein, and the presence of a small amount of fat. If you really can't live without your sweets, then skip to the end of the list of snacks for indulgent desserts.

Top Snacks of Choice

Greek Yogurt
Almonds
Nut Butters
Cheese
Berries
Apple
Banana
Big Train Fit Frappe Protein Powder
EAS Low-Carb Advantage Shake
Muscle Milk Light
Veggies & Hummus
Air-popped Popcorn
Hard-boiled Eggs

Fruit, Nuts, & Yogurt

1 Medium Chocolate Covered Strawberry 23
EAS Low Carb-Advantage Protein Shake 120
Total Calories 143

4 Medium Chocolate Covered Strawberries 92

8 Large Organic Strawberries 46
Sugar-Free Chocolate Pudding cup 60
Total Calories 106

Yoplait Delights Chocolate Raspberry Parfait 100
10 Organic Raspberries 10
Total Calories 110

6 oz. of Melon, fresh (on Avg.) 60
Yoplait Honey Vanilla Nonfat Greek Yogurt 100
Total Calories 160

1 Medium Organic Apple 95
2 tsp. Natural Creamy Peanut Butter 59
Total Calories 154

1 cup Pineapple, fresh 83
1 wedge Laughing Cow Light Swiss Cheese 35
Total Calories 118

1 Small Pear 81
6 Praline Pecans 85
Total Calories 166

7 Almonds, raw 49
Flavored Nonfat Yogurt (on Avg. 6 oz.) 100
Total Calories 149

Yoplait Delights Crème Caramel 100
1/2 Medium Organic Apple 47
Total Calories 147

Yoplait Honey Vanilla Nonfat Greek Yogurt 100
1/2 cup Organic Blueberries 41
Total Calories 141

0.5 oz. of 70% Cacao Dark Chocolate 78
1 Clementine 35
Total Calories 113

1 Medium Banana (about 4.2 oz.) 105
1 tsp. Natural Creamy Peanut Butter 31
Total Calories 136

2 cups of Water Melon 92 Calories

1 Large Banana (about 4.8 oz.) 121
4 Almonds, raw 28
Total Calories 149

8 Cherries, fresh 41
0.5 oz. of 70% Cacao Dark Chocolate 78
Total Calories 119

1 cup Grapes 104

½ cup Grapes 52
½ oz. Goat Cheese, crumbles 40
5 Candied Pecans, chopped 45
Total Calories 137

1 cup Organic Mixed Berries, Frozen 70
2 Tbsp. Cool Whip Free 15
Total Calories 85

1 Medium Plum (3.5 oz.) 45 Calories

1 Large Peach (6 oz.) 65
2 Tbsp. Cool Whip Free 15
1 tsp. Cinnamon
Total Calories 80

Veggies & Dips

1/2 cup Cucumber, raw with peel 8
1 oz. Feta, Crumbled 75
1/2 cup Cherry Tomatoes, fresh, raw 13
1 Tbsp. Reduced Fat Italian Dressing 11
Total Calories 107

1 cup Cauliflower, raw (3.5 oz.) 25
3 oz. Baby Carrots, raw 30
2 Tbsp. Reduced-Fat Ranch Dressing or Greek Yogurt Veggie Dip 60
Total Calories 115

1 cup Chopped Broccoli, raw (3.2 oz.) 31
1 cup Cauliflower, Raw (3.5 oz.) 25
2 Tbsp. Reduced-Fat Ranch Dressing or Greek Yogurt Veggie Dip 60
(I like Marzetti's Otria Greek Yogurt Veggie Dip.)
Total Calories 116

3 oz. Baby Carrots, raw 30
1 Medium 12" Celery Stalk 9
2 Tbsp. Reduced-Fat Ranch Dressing or Greek Yogurt Veggie Dip 60
Total Calories 99

3 oz. Baby Carrots, raw 30
1 Medium 12" Celery Stalk 9
2 Tbsp. Hummus 50
Total Calories 89

1 Small Whole Wheat Pita (4" diameter, 1 oz.) 74
2 Tbsp. Hummus 50
1/2 Large Red or Yellow Pepper 21
Total Calories 145

1 Medium 12" Celery Stalk 9
1 Tbsp. Creamy Natural Peanut Butter 90
Total Calories 99

1 Medium 12" Celery Stalk 9
2 Tbsp. Whipped Cream Cheese 70
Total Calories 79

2 Jalapenos 8
Stuffed with the following:
2 Tbsp. Whipped Cream Cheese 70
1 Tbsp. Chopped Bacon Cooked Crisp 25
Bake at 350 degrees for 12 minutes.
Total Calories 103

10 Edamame Pods, boiled 30
2 oz. Smoked Salmon 66
1 Tbsp. Soy Sauce for dipping 11
Wasabi Powder or Paste 1
Total Calories 108

2 oz. Roast Beef Deli Meat 90
1 tsp. Horseradish, jar 2
1 Tbsp. Light Mayo 35
4 Asparagus Spears, blanched 13
Total Calories 140

Salt Craving

100-calorie package of Microwave Popcorn

8 Tortilla Chips 105
2 Tbsp. Tostitos Salsa Con Queso, jar 40
Total Calories 145

12 Tortilla Chips 140
2 Tbsp. Salsa (on Avg.) 15
Total Calories 155

20 Baked Kettle Chips, Assorted Flavors 120 Calories

17 to 18 Pop Chips, Assorted Flavors 100 Calories

1 oz. Baked Ruffles, Plain 120 Calories

1 oz. Rold Gold Classic Tiny Twists Pretzels 110 Calories

24 Glutino Gluten-free Pretzel Twists 120 Calories

Cheese Please!

1 Whole Wheat Mini Bagel 120
1 Tbsp. Whipped Cream Cheese 35
Total Calories 155

1 wedge Laughing Cow Light Cheese, Assorted Flavors 35
16 Reduced-fat Wheat Thins 130
Total Calories 165

1 Mini Babybel Light 50
1 Medium Organic Apple 95
Total Calories 145

1 Mini Babybel Light 50
1 cup Grapes 104
Total Calories 154

1 Stick 2% Mozzarella String Cheese 70
½ cup Grapes 52
Total Calories 122

1 oz. Cheddar Cheese 110
8 Glutino Gluten-free Pretzels 40
Total Calories 150

Desserts

150-Calorie Mocha Protein Pudding

My go-to, delightfully decadent, sinless dessert is Mocha Protein Pudding. It is low-calorie, high-fiber (5.5g), and high-protein. You could also try this with another flavor from Fit Frappe like chocolate or vanilla.

Ingredients
2 scoops (1/2 cup) Big Train Fit Frappe Mocha Protein Powder
1/2 cup Original Almond Milk

Directions
Combine the ingredients in a blender and serve.

Number of Servings: 1

Nutrition Information/Serving:

Calories: 150
Fat: 5g
Carbohydrates: 26g
Protein: 21g

Betty Crocker Warm Delights Minis Molten Chocolate Cake 150

Betty Crocker Warm Delights Minis Molten Caramel Cake 150

Betty Crocker Warm Delights Minis Decadent Dark Chocolate 150

Enjoy Life Soft Baked Cookies (2), Assorted Flavors 120

Kashi Cookie, Assorted Flavors 130

Skinny Cow Ice Cream Snack cups, Assorted Flavors 150 to 170

Skinny Cow Ice Cream Sandwiches, Assorted Flavors 140 to 160

Skinny Cow Ice Cream Cones, Assorted Flavors 150

Skinny Cow Ice Cream Bars, Assorted Flavors 100

Skinny Cow Mini Fudge Pops 40

Smart Ones Smart Delights Brownie A La Mode 130

Smart Ones Smart Delights Chocolate Chip Cookie Dough Sundae 140

Smart Ones Smart Delights Chocolate Fudge Brownie Sundae 140

Smart Ones Smart Delights Key Lime Pie 150

Smart Ones Smart Delights Peanut Butter cup Sundae 140

Smart Ones Smart Delights Strawberry Shortcake 120

Smart Ones Smart Delights Turtle Sundae 140

Dinner

For dinner I have set the calorie budget at 500 to 650 calories. That may seem like a difficult target to hit when dining out, because a lot of restaurant dinners are more like 1,000 calories or more. To simplify dining out I have scaled down the restaurant menus to help you make better choices. Many of the menus allow you to choose your own sides. Limit starches to only one side, and choose a green vegetable for your second side. Avoid alcoholic beverages and stick to water or unsweetened iced tea.

Many of the dinners at home are significantly less than 500 to 650 calories. This will allow you to make a great choice at dinner if you feel like you went overboard at lunch. If you are on target for the day, then maybe you can indulge a little bit more at dinner with a caloric beverage or a dessert from the snack menu. Just be careful not to overdo it.

Sit-Down Dining

Applebee's

Have it All - includes sides
Napa Chicken & Portobellos 490
Savory Cedar Salmon 520
Thai Shrimp Salad 380
Steakhouse Bruschetta Sirloin 530
Pepper Crusted Sirloin & Whole Grains 350
Cedar Grilled Lemon Chicken 560
Shrimp & Broccoli Cavatappi 450

Bob Evans

Just as I noted earlier in the breakfast section, Bob Evans has a Fit From the Farm Menu so I have listed those menu items first. There are also a few additional low-calorie options on the regular menu so I have listed those options separately.

Fit From the Farm Menu
Slow-Roasted Chicken-N-Noodles 116
Grilled Chicken Breast with Baked Potato & Broccoli Florets 413
Potato Crusted Flounder with Baked Potato & Broccoli Florets 442
Grilled Salmon Fillet with Baked Potato & Broccoli Florets 509
Apple-Cranberry Spinach Salad w/Reduced-fat Raspberry Dressing 372

Savor Size Apple-Cranberry Spinach Salad w/Reduced-fat Raspberry Dressing 364
Cup of Beef Vegetable Soup 93
Cup of Bean Soup 127

Regular Menu Savor Size Entrée's
Savor Size Chicken & Broccoli Alfredo 451
Savor Size Pot Roast Stroganoff 431
Savor Size Spaghetti with Meat Sauce 468
Regular Menu Savor Size Salads (pair with a 1.6 oz. serving of one of the following dressings: Lite Ranch 110, Balsamic Vinaigrette 59, Wildfire Ranch 129, or Reduced-fat Raspberry Vinaigrette 114.)
Savor Size Cobb Salad 300
Savor Size Heritage Chef Salad 197
Savor Size Wildfire Grilled Chicken Salad 236
Savor Size Cranberry Pecan Chicken Salad 499

Boston Market

Boston Market is technically fast food, which makes it a great option for a high-protein meal when you are in a bit of a time crunch. Rotisserie chicken is delicious, flavorful, and packed with protein. Just make sure you pull off the skin to reduce the fat/calorie content of your meal. They also offer turkey breast and beef brisket.

Individual Meals (Sides not included.)
Rotisserie Chicken – Quarter White 320
Rotisserie Chicken – Quarter White, No Skin 220
Rotisserie Chicken – 3-Piece Dark, No Skin, Thigh, 2 Drumsticks 280
Rotisserie Chicken – 1 Thigh, 1 Drumstick 310
Turkey Breast – Large 260
Turkey Breast – Regular 180
Beef Brisket – Regular 230
Meatloaf – Regular 480

Gourmet Sides
Mediterranean Green Beans 120
Garlicky Lemon Spinach 140
Mashed Potatoes w/o gravy 300
Sweet Corn 170
Garlic Dill New Potatoes 140
Fresh Steamed Vegetables 60
Fresh Vegetable Stuffing 190
Green Beans (regional) 60
Cornbread 180

Half Sandwiches (Pair with Half Salad, Soup, or Side.)

Rotisserie Chicken Carver – Half 380
Hand Carved Turkey Carver – Half 395
Brisket Dip Carver – Half 420
Homestyle Meatloaf Carver – Half 470
Pulled BBQ Rotisserie Chicken – Half 345
All White Rotisserie Chicken Salad – Half 525

Salads & Soups

Mediterranean – Half Salad 320
Southwest Santa Fe – Half Salad 370
Caesar Salad – Half Salad 330
Chicken Noodle Soup 240

Sauces

Au Jus 20
Zesty Barbecue (mild) 60
Sweet Thai Chili Garlic (medium hot) 60
Honey Habanero (medium hot) 60
Beef Gravy 10
Poultry Gravy 10

California Pizza Kitchen

Small Plates
Spicy Chicken Tinga Quesadilla 460
Asparagus & Arugula Salad 180
Petite Wedge 280
Bianco Flatbread 380
Shaved Mushroom & Spinach Flatbread 400
Spicy Fennel Sausage & Poblano Flatbread 390

Appetizers
Lettuce Wraps with Chicken 610
Lettuce Wraps with Shrimp 480
Sesame Ginger Chicken Dumplings 370

Soups
Artichoke & Broccoli Soup Bowl 200, cup 100
Sedona Tortilla Soup Bowl 480, cup 260
Dakota Smashed Pea & Barley Soup Bowl 340, cup 170

Half Salads (Fat-Free Vinaigrette available on request, 110 calories per 1.5 oz.)
BBQ Chicken Chopped Half Salad, No Avocado 550
Caramelized Peach Half Salad 450
Caramelized Peach Half Salad with Grilled Shrimp 510
Roasted Vegetable Half Salad 360
Roasted Vegetable Half Salad with Grilled Chicken Breast 550

Roasted Vegetable Half Salad with Grilled Shrimp 420

Roasted Vegetable Half Salad with Sautéed Salmon 680

CPK Cobb Half Salad with Ranch Dressing 450

CPK Cobb Half Salad with Ranch Dressing & Beets 470

CPK Cobb Half Salad with Blue Cheese Dressing 520

Classic Caesar Half Salad 270

Classic Caesar Half Salad with Grilled Chicken Breast 460

Classic Caesar Half Salad with Grilled Shrimp 320

Classic Caesar Half Salad with Sautéed Salmon 590

Chinese Chicken Half Salad 420

Thai Crunch Half Salad, No Avocado 650

Italian Chopped Half Salad 490

Waldorf Chicken Half Salad 610

Pizza

If you cannot fathom going to California Pizza Kitchen without ordering pizza, then stick with eating only HALF of the thin crust pizza. You can split it with a friend or take the rest home as leftovers.

Half Roasted Artichoke & Spinach Thin Crust Pizza 555

Half Roasted Artichoke & Spinach Thin Crust Pizza with Chicken 605

Half Jamaican Jerk Chicken Thin Crust Pizza 625

Half Margherita Thin Crust Pizza 665

Chili's Grill & Bar

Salads (Dressing included unless otherwise indicated.)
Caribbean Salad with Grilled Chicken 610
Caribbean Salad with Grilled Shrimp 590
House Salad No Dressing 150
Dressing, Honey Mustard No Fat 70
Dressing, Low Fat Ranch 80

Soups (without crackers)
Chicken Enchilada Bowl 380, cup 190
Chili's Terlingua Chili with Toppings Bowl 360, cup 180
Loaded Baked Potato Soup Bowl 410, cup 210
Southwest Chicken & Sausage Bowl 330, cup 160

Lighter Choices (as served)
Classic Sirloin w/Grilled Avocado 410
Grilled Chicken Salad 430
Ancho Salmon 600
Mango-Chile Chicken or Tilapia 520
Margarita Grilled Chicken 580

Not "Just" Sides
Black Beans 100
Black Bean Patty Only 200
Rice 190
Steamed Broccoli 80
Sweet Corn on the Cob with Butter 200

Longhorn Steakhouse

There are several options for eating low-calorie at Longhorn. You may start with one of the side salads and order soup as your main course. You might opt for one of their lower-calorie entrée salads. If you choose a protein-packed entrée, then stick with one of the leaner entrees that I have suggested. Keep in mind that it comes with a salad and a side. The lowest calorie salad is the mixed green side salad (100 calories) with fat-free ranch dressing (45 calories). Skip the starchy sides and order green vegetables. If you are craving the loaded baked potato (440 calories) or the sweet potato (380), then order it as your entrée. Be strong and skip the bread loaf (510 calories) so that you don't break the calorie bank. Try not to go over 650 calories with your order combination. There is nothing wrong with getting a box for leftovers. If you enjoy your meal, then you can enjoy it twice!

Soups
Mushroom Truffle Bisque 280
French Onion Soup (bowl) 380
Shrimp & Lobster Chowder (bowl) 250
Loaded Baked Potato Soup (bowl) 380

Dinner Entrees - Salads
Grilled Chicken & Strawberry Salad w/Vinaigrette 530
7-Pepper Sirloin Salad 490

Dinner Entrees – Legendary Steaks
Flo's Fillet 6 oz. 370
Renegade Sirloin 6 oz. 320
Flat Iron Steak 8 oz. 430
Flo's Fillet & Lobster Tail 6 oz. 460

Dinner Entrees – Seafood
Longhorn Salmon 7 oz. 300
Redrock Grilled Shrimp 240

Dinner Entrees – Chicken
Napa Grilled Chicken 530
Spinach Feta Chicken 360

Dinner Entrees – Light & Flavorful
Grilled Fresh Tilapia with Mango Salsa 570
Balsamic-Raspberry Seared Chicken 450
Rosemary Cabernet Filet 280

Ribs, Chops & More
Cowboy Pork Chops 400

Side Dishes
Fresh Steamed Broccoli 90
Fresh Green Beans 30
Mixed Green Side Salad 100
Caesar Side Salad with Caesar Dressing 280
Fresh Grilled Asparagus 90
Mashed Potatoes 340
Parmesan Mushroom Risotto 360

Olive Garden

The key at Olive Garden is to either order an appetizer/soup, salad, and a breadstick or simply order the entrée without all the accoutrements. While many of the entrees at Olive Garden break the 650-calorie budget that I have allotted for dinner, I have listed the few entrees that actually hit the range. For those entrees that listed that exceed the budget only eat half the entrée, and start with a soup or salad.

Appetizers
Breadstick (with garlic-butter spread) 140
Stuffed Mushrooms 380

Soups & Salads
Chicken & Gnocchi (one serving) 250
Pasta e Fagioli (one serving) 180
Minestrone (one serving) 100
Zuppa Toscana (one serving) 220
Garden-Fresh Salad (one serving) 140

Lighter Fare Dinner Entrees
Chicken Abruzzi 540
Center Cut Filet Mignon 360
Garlic Rosemary Chicken 550
Baked Tilapia with Shrimp 360
Citrus Chicken Sorrento 530
Herb-Grilled Salmon 470

Dinner Entrees

(Only eat half the entrée, and take the rest home.)

Steak Toscano 840

Ravioli di Portobello 810

Cheese Ravioli with Marinara Sauce 770

Salmon Bruschetta 860

Baked Parmesan Shrimp 860

Parmesan Crusted Filet 710

On the Border

When ordering Mexican food it can be difficult to stay under 650 calories for dinner. I would suggest skipping the high-calorie margaritas and the chips and dips. If your entrée comes with beans and rice, then box them up for a later meal. If it is available, then order a la carte. There are a few options at On the Border that make the cut.

Soup & Salads
Chicken Tortilla Soup Bowl 470, cup 290
Mango Chicken Salad with Mango Citrus Vinaigrette 400
Side – House Salad without Dressing 160

Create Your Own Combo (listed without rice & beans) Pick two.
Chicken Tortilla Soup 290
Crispy Taco – Chicken 260
Crispy Taco – Ground Beef 320
Enchilada – Chicken with Sour Cream Sauce 200
Enchilada – Green Chile Chicken 170
Enchilada – Ground Beef with Chile con Carne 250
Enchilada – Spinach & Mushroom with Sour Cream Sauce 190
Side – House Salad without Dressing 160
Soft Taco – Chicken 270
Tostadas – Chicken 140
Tostadas – Ground Beef 180
Tostadas – Guacamole 200

Fajita Grill (listed w/o rice, condiments, & beans)
Chicken Fajitas 320
Grilled Vegetable Fajitas 240
Sautéed Shrimp Fajitas 410
Steak Fajitas 420
Stick to only one starch: tortillas, beans, or rice. Skip the flour tortillas (360 for 3) and opt for the corn tortillas (150 for 3). Black beans are a better choice (170) over refried beans (210) and Mexican rice (280). The condiments served with the fajitas aren't too bad, but they can add up:
Guacamole 45
Mixed Cheese 110
Pico de Gallo 10
Sour Cream 60

Fresh Grill (listed as served.)
Jalapeno-BBQ Salmon 570

Outback Steakhouse

Skip the Bread & Butter! It's listed on the nutrition facts as 314 calories. If you can't resist it, then just have one small slice of bread and a cup of soup. My favorite low-cal option is to pair a high-protein entrée with fresh vegetables and seasoned rice for a nutrient-rich meal.

Appetizers
Grilled Shrimp on the Barbie 291
Gold Coast Coconut Shrimp 458
Seared Ahi Tuna (small) 362

Daily Soups
Potato Soup Bowl 588, cup 413
Chicken Tortilla Soup Bowl 219, cup 174
White Bean Sausage Soup Bowl 442, cup 295
Creamy Onion Soup Bowl 482, cup 329
Clam Chowder Bowl 570, cup 386
Too Right French Onion Soup 465

Freshly Made Salads
Shrimp Caesar Salad (Dressing included) 564
Ahi Tuna Chopped Salad Small (Dressing included) 334
Aussie Chicken Cobb Salad Grilled (Dressing not included) 509
Queensland Salad Small (Dressing not included) 461

Dressing
Tangy Tomato Dressing – 3 oz. 111
Tangy Tomato Dressing – 1.5 oz. 55
Wasabi Vinaigrette Dressing – 1.5 oz. 132

Outback Favorites (Sides not included.)
Chicken on the Barbie Regular 305
Chicken on the Barbie Small 190
Filet with Wild Mushroom Sauce 406
Sweet Glazed Pork Tenderloin 300
Wood-Fire Grilled Pork Chop (1) 381

Signature Steaks (Sides not included.)
Outback Special – 6oz. 254
Victoria's Filet – 6oz. 218
Prime Rib – 8 oz. (with Au Jus) 479

Wood-Fire Grilled Steaks (Sides not included.)
Outback Special – 6 oz. 246
Victoria's Filet – 6 oz. 228
Prime Rib – 8 oz. (with Au Jus) 501

Add On Mates
Wild Mushroom Sauce 102
Barbeque Sauce 63
Cabernet Wine Sauce 64
Au Jus 7

Perfect Combinations (Sides not included.)
6 oz. Sirloin with Grilled Shrimp 505
6 oz. Sirloin & Coconut Shrimp 512

Straight from the Sea (Sides not included.)
Norwegian Salmon 387
Simply Grilled Tilapia 227
Lobster 4 oz. – 2 Tails 448
Simply Grilled Mahi 292

Burgers and Sandwiches (Sides not included.)
G'Day Fish Sandwich 513
Chicken Club Sandwich 510

Freshly Made Sides
Fresh Seasonal Veggies 96
Fresh Steamed Broccoli 109
Seasoned Rice 129
House Salad w/Tangy Tomato Dressing 216

Order these sides as your entrée. Pair with a side or cup of soup.
Garlic Mashed Potatoes 305
Baked Potato with Butter and Sour Cream 314
Baked Potato with Everything 358
Sweet Potato (plain) 318
Sweet Potato w/Honey Butter 418
Sweet Potato w/Brown Sugar 364
Caesar Salad (Dressing included) 332
Classic Blue Cheese Wedge Salad (Dressing included) 428
House Salad w/Ranch Dressing 378

Papa Murphy's

I love Papa Murphy's Take 'N Bake Pizza! It's fresh and easy. Plus they offer gluten-free crust at select locations.

For portion-control, I find it helpful to think of pizza as an open-faced sandwich. In other words, think of 1 slice of thin crust pizza as a half sandwich and 2 slices as a whole sandwich. One slice of the original crust is more like a whole sandwich so stick with the thin crust pizza.

Start with a serving of salad to make it a balanced meal. While it may be tempting to eat half the pizza try to remind yourself that's like eating two whole sandwiches in one sitting. Save the second helping for lunch the following day.

Salads (Start with 1 serving = ½ salad, dressing and croutons not included.)

Caesar Salad 50
Chicken Caesar Salad 110
Club Salad 140
Garden Salad 96
Italian Salad 132
Mediterranean Salad 191
Croutons (1/2 Packet) 45

Dressing (1/2 Packet)

Balsamic Vinaigrette 70

Buttermilk Ranch Salad Dressing 120
Low-calorie Italian Salad Dressing 15
Thousand Island Salad Dressing 120

Large Size Thin Crust Pizzas - 1 Serving = 1 Slice = 1/8th of the Pizza
All Meat 239
Barbeque Chicken 229
Cheese 178
Chicken Bacon Ranch 248
Chicken Pesto 226
Chicken Garlic 220
Classic Italian 249
Cowboy 238
Gourmet Angus Steak & Roasted Garlic 217
Gourmet Chicken Bacon Artichoke 235
Gourmet Spicy Sausage 241
Gourmet Vegetarian 208
Hawaiian 197
Herb Chicken Mediterranean 224
Murphy's Combo 250
Papa's Favorite 242
Pepperoni 213
Rancher 221
Specialty of the House 217
Taco Grande (Beef) 211
Taco Grande (Chicken) 208
Thai Chicken 228
Garden Veggie 195

Medium Gluten Free Crust Pizzas - 1 Serving = 1 Slice = 1/8th of the Pizza
All Meat 278
Barbeque Chicken 268
Cheese 218
Chicken Bacon Artichoke 275
Chicken Bacon Ranch 287
Chicken Garlic 259
Cowboy 274
Gourmet Vegetarian 248
Hawaiian 236
Herb Chicken Mediterranean 264
Murphy's Combo 289
Papa's Favorite 282
Pepperoni 252
Rancher 260
Specialty of the House 256
Taco Grande (Beef) 250
Taco Grande (Chicken) 247
Thai Chicken 268
Garden Veggie 235

Large Size The Faves Line Pizzas - 1 Serving = 1 Slice = 1/8th of the Pizza
Cheese Fave 218
Pepperoni Fave 240
Pepperoni & Sausage Fave 259

Red Lobster

Seaside Starters (Sauces/Sides not included.)
Parrot Isle Jumbo Coconut Shrimp 510
Chilled Jumbo Shrimp Cocktail 100
Crispy Shrimp Lettuce Wraps 620

Soups and Salads (Sauces/Sides not included.)
New England Clam Chowder Bowl 400, cup 200
Creamy Potato Bacon Soup Bowl 510, cup 250
Lobster Bisque Bowl 570, cup 290
Classic Caesar Salad 540
Classic Caesar Salad w/Shrimp 640
Manhattan Clam Chowder Bowl 160, cup 80
Seafood Gumbo Bowl 350, cup 170

Add to Any Meal (Sauces/Sides not included.)
Maine Lobster Tail 90
Garlic-Grilled Jumbo Shrimp Skewer 60
Snow Crab Legs (1/2 pound) 90

Create Your Own Combination (Sauces/Sides not included.)
Garlic-Grilled Shrimp 230
Seafood-Stuffed Flounder 170
Wood-Grilled Fresh Salmon 280
Garlic Shrimp Scampi 150
Steamed Snow Crab Legs 90
Peppercorn-Grilled Sirloin 240

Grilled Selections (Sauces/Sides not included.)
Grilled Lobster, Shrimp, and Scallops 500
Garlic-Grilled Jumbo Shrimp 370
Peach-Bourbon BBQ Shrimp and Scallops 490
Center-Cut NY Strip Steak 490

Lobster and Crab (Sauces/Sides not included.)
Ultimate Feast 650
Snow Crab Legs (1 pound, includes corn, potatoes) 370
Rock Lobster Tail 170
Live Maine Lobster (includes corn, potatoes) 350
Live Maine Lobster Steamed 420
Live Maine Lobster w/Stuffing 500

Shrimp (Sauces/Sides not included.)
Shrimp Linguini Alfredo Half Order 630
Shrimp Your Way:
Scampi 100
Fried Shrimp 220

Fish (Sauces/Sides not included.)
Tilapia with Roasted Vegetables 540
Parmesan-Crusted Tilapia 370
Seafood-Stuffed Flounder/Sole 330
Flounder/Sole Oven-Broiled 340
Flounder/Sole Golden-Fried 500
Walleye Blackened 440
Walleye Broiled 400

Accompaniments, Condiments, and Sauces

Cheddar Bay Biscuit (each) 160
Garden Salad 70
Caesar Salad 270
Balsamic Vinaigrette – 1.5 oz. 80
Caesar Dressing - 1.5 oz. 280
Coleslaw 260
Fresh Broccoli 50
Petite Green Beans 90
Home-Style Mashed Potatoes 210
Wild Rice Pilaf 170
Fresh Asparagus 60
Lemon Wedge 5

Dipping Sauces – 1.5 oz.

100% Pure Melted Butter 300
Cocktail Sauce 45
Honey Mustard Dipping Sauce 190
Ketchup 60
Marinara Sauce 35
Pico de Gallo 10
Pineapple Salsa 40
Pina Colada Sauce 100
Tartar Sauce 210

Ruby Tuesday's

One thing I love about Ruby Tuesday's is that the restaurant offers some delicious low-calorie sides. In addition they have a Fit & Trim menu offering. The Fit & Trim items are less than 700 calories when served with Roasted Spaghetti Squash and Fresh Grilled Zucchini. Note that the nutrition information listed does not include sauces that may be served with your entrée.

Fit & Trim Choices w/Squash and Zucchini
Petite Sirloin 379
Top Sirloin 443
Hickory Bourbon Chicken 355
Chicken Bella 426
Grilled Salmon 425
Hickory Bourbon Salmon 485

More Fit & Trim Choices
Fresh Grilled Zucchini 41
Fresh Green Beans 68
Fresh Steamed Broccoli 52
Roasted Spaghetti Squash 54

Soups
Broccoli Cheese Soup 325
Chicken Noodle Soup 180
Chicken Tortilla Soup 166

Premium Seafood *(Sides not included.)*
Hickory Bourbon Salmon 390
Crab Cake Dinner 170
Grilled Salmon 330
Jumbo Skewered Shrimp 274
Herb-Crusted Tilapia 401
New Orleans Seafood 317

Steakhouse Steaks *(Sides not included.)*
Petite Sirloin 284
Petite Sirloin and Lobster Tail 397
Petite Sirloin and Coconut-Crusted Shrimp 418
Top Sirloin 349
Asiago Peppercorn Sirloin 373

Fresh All-Natural Chicken *(Sides not included.)*
Chicken Fresco 352
Chicken Bella 332
Hickory Bourbon Chicken 250

Dressings & Condiments per oz.
Hickory Bourbon Barbecue Sauce 60
Balsamic Vinaigrette Dressing 40
BBQ Sauce 60
Cocktail Sauce 23
Lemon Butter Sauce 87
Lite Ranch Dressing 70
Parmesan Cream Sauce 58
Siracha Ranch 75

T.G.I. Friday's

All items are listed as served unless otherwise indicated.

Appetizers, Taste & Share (Order as a meal.)
Thai Pork Tacos 280
Ahi Tuna Crisps 330
Hibachi Skewers – Black Angus Sirloin 490
Hibachi Skewers – Grilled Chicken 470
Spinach Florentine Flatbread 540
BBQ Chicken Flatbread 620

Seafood
Grilled Salmon with Langostino Lobster (add sides) 540

Salads
Balsamic-Glazed Chicken Caesar 500
Classic Wedge Salad 620
House Salad w/Breadstick (add choice of dressing) 210
Caesar Salad w/Breadstick 270
Smart Choice Salad Dressing per 2 oz. Serving
Low Fat Balsamic Vinaigrette 80

Soups (Order as a meal or pair with a side salad.)
French Onion 310
White Cheddar Broccoli Cheese 290
Soup of the Day – New England Clam Chowder 500
Soup of the Day – Tortilla 250

Soup of the Day – Chicken Noodle 250
Soup of the Day – Tomato Basil 300

Jack Daniel's Grill (Add choice of sides.)
Flat Iron 500
Chicken & Shrimp 530
Chicken 540

Signature Sides (If you order a starch choose broccoli as 2nd side.)
Fresh Broccoli 50
Fresh Spinach 180
Ginger-Lime Slaw 80
Mashed Potatoes 210
Tomato Mozzarella Salad 110

Dinner at Home

Fish

Oven-Fried Fish
1 Fillet Battered Fish, frozen, baked 200
10 Popcorn Shrimp 130
2 Tbsp. Cocktail Sauce or Ketchup 40
½ Amy's Frozen Entrée Macaroni & Cheese 200
1 cup steamed broccoli 20
Total Calories 590

Blackened Mahi Mahi
4 oz. Mahi Mahi Fillet, baked in foil pack 96
Season with Blackened Seasoning (or sub Old Bay Seasoning)
& Top with 1 slice fresh Pineapple (0.5" thick) 28
½ cup long grain white rice, cooked 103
¾ cup Birds Eye Steamfresh California Medley 30
Total Calories 257

Fish Tacos & Spicy Brown Rice

Tortilla Crusted Tilapia Fillet, frozen, baked (3.5 oz.) 200

2 soft corn tortillas or 1 flour taco size tortilla 110

¼ cup Shredded Cabbage mixed with 5

1 tsp. Spicy Ranch Dressing (optional) 25

1 Tbsp. Pico de Gallo or Salsa 10

Lime Wedge or Lemon Wedge 3

¼ cup Black Beans 55

Spicy Brown Rice (1/4 Recipe, which follows) 114

Total Calories 522

Spicy Brown Rice

Ingredients

2 cups chicken broth or water

2 roasted poblano peppers, stems, seeds and skin removed

1 jalapeno pepper, stem, seeds and rib removed, finely diced (optional)

1/2 cup chopped fresh cilantro leaves, divided

1 tablespoon vegetable oil

1 white onion, finely diced

4 garlic cloves, peeled and finely chopped

1 cup brown long-grain rice (can sub white rice or quinoa)

Salt to taste

Directions

Heat the broth in a medium saucepan over medium heat. Puree the roasted poblano chilies in a food processor or blender with a little bit of the broth. Add 1/4 cup cilantro and process to a smooth puree. Season with salt. Stir the puree into the broth. Increase the heat, bring to a boil, and then partially cover and simmer gently over medium-low heat while you prepare the rice.

In a separate medium sauce pan, add the oil, and heat over medium-high heat. Add the onions and cook until soft. Add the garlic and jalapeno. Cook for 1 minute. Stir in the rice and cook for 1 minute. Add the warm broth mixture, stir, and season with salt. If the broth has reduced quite a bit, then add some water. Bring to a boil, cover, and then reduce the heat to medium-low and cook for 15 minutes. Remove from the heat and let sit for 5 minutes, covered. Fluff with a fork, transfer to a bowl, and stir in remaining cilantro.

Number of Servings: 4

Nutrition Information/Serving:

Calories: 114
Fat: 4g
Carbohydrates: 17g
Protein: 3g

Easy Breaded Tilapia & Lemon Caper Mayo
Frozen Breaded Tilapia Fillet, baked (3.5 oz.) 200
1 cup Broccoli, chopped, steamed 20
1/2 cup long grain white rice, cooked 103
2 Tbsp. Lemon Caper Mayo, recipe follows 71
Total 394

Lemon Caper Mayo

Ingredients
1 Tbsp. Capers
½ cup Light Mayonnaise
1/2 tsp. Lemon Juice (fresh squeezed)
1/4 tsp. Ground Black Pepper

Directions
Chop the capers fine and mix all the ingredients together. Serve immediately. Pepper to taste.

Servings: 3

Nutrition Information/Serving:

Calories: 71
Fat: 7g
Carbohydrates: 2g
Protein: 0g

Crab Cakes

Ingredients
1 Can of Crab Meat, preferably Lump, drained
10 Saltine Crackers, crushed
1 Tbsp. Spicy Brown Mustard
2 tsp. Worcestershire Sauce
1 Egg White, beaten
1 Tbsp. of Shallot, finally diced
1.5 Tbsp. of Extra Virgin Olive Oil
2 tsp. Dried dill
½ tsp. Old Bay Seasoning
1 tsp. Paprika
1/2 tsp. Cayenne pepper, or more to taste
Salt and Pepper to taste

Directions
Preheat the oven at 350 degrees.

Heat 1/2 tbsp. of olive oil on the stove on medium high heat. Once the oil starts to smoke toss in the diced shallot. Salt and pepper the shallot and cook for 1 minute.

Combine the shallot with the crab, crushed saltines, mustard, egg white, and spices. Go easy on the salt because the saltines are already salty.

Heat 1 tbsp. of olive oil in the skillet on medium high heat. While waiting for that to heat up create 2 patties out the crab mixture each about 1/2 cup. I like to use the measuring cup to form the patty. Once the oil starts to smoke add the crab cakes to the skillet. Cook them on each side for 2 1/2 to 3 minutes. Transfer the crab cakes to the oven and cook for an additional 15 minutes. Serve immediately over a lightly dressed salad.

Number of Servings: 2, each about 1/2 cup

Nutrition Information/Serving:

Calories: 230
Fat: 13g
Carbohydrates: 14g
Protein: 15g

Notice: Consuming raw or undercooked meats, poultry, seafood, shellfish, or eggs may increase your risk of food-borne illness, especially if you have certain medical conditions.

Poultry

Easy Chicken Fettuccine Alfredo
4 oz. Rotisserie Chicken Breast w/o skin 138
1/2 cup peas 62
1/2 cup Fettuccine pasta, cooked 180
1/4 cup Bertolli Mushroom Alfredo Sauce 80
2 tsp. Grated Parmesan 20
Total Calories 480

Pesto Chicken & Dumplings
Rotisserie Chicken Breast No Skin (4.9 oz.) 170
3/4 cup Potato Gnocchetti or Gnocchi 170
½ cup Chicken Broth 5
1 oz. Bertolli Brand Pesto 135
Cook the gnocchi according to package instructions. Heat up the chicken broth and pesto in a sauce pan. Combine everything in the sauce pan once the gnocchi is cooked.
Total Calories 480

Rotisserie Chicken & Cheesy Mashed Cauliflower

4 oz. Rotisserie Chicken Breast w/o skin 138
1/2 cup Cheesy Mashed Cauliflower, recipe follows
97
1 cup Broccoli, Steamed 20
Protein Pudding (see page 105) 150
10 Medium Strawberries, fresh 38
Total Calories 443

Cheesy Mashed Cauliflower

Ingredients

1 Large or 2 Small Heads of Cauliflower, chopped
2 Tbsp. Whipped Cream Cheese
2 Tbsp. Parmesan Cheese, Grated
1/2 cup 5-Cheese Italian Blend, Shredded
1 tsp. Minced Garlic, from a jar (optional)
Salt to taste

Directions

Steam the cauliflower covered for 8 minutes or until tender over medium high heat.

While the cauliflower is cooking, mix the remaining ingredients in a separate mixing bowl.

Salt the steamed cauliflower to taste. Slowly add the cauliflower to a food processor or blender, while mixing to desired consistency.
Add the cheese mixture to the processor and pulse a few times. Transfer to a serving bowl.

Number of Servings: 6

Nutrition Information/Serving:

Calories: 97
Fat: 4g
Total Carbs: 11g
Protein: 7g

Beef

Beef Tenderloin & Mushroom Gorgonzola Soup
4 oz. Grilled Filet Mignon 202
¾ cup Gorgonzola Mushroom Soup, recipe follows 276
1 cup Steamed Green Beans, fresh 44
Total Calories 522

Mushroom Gorgonzola Soup

Ingredients
1 Tbsp. of Butter, unsalted
1 Tbsp. of Olive Oil
1 package Green Giant Gourmet mix of mushrooms
1 large Shallot, diced
1 Tbsp. Garlic
1 oz. of Port or Cooking Sherry (optional)
1 tsp. of dried Thyme
1 cup of Half & Half
2 cups of Milk, 2%
1/2 cup of Gorgonzola Crumbles
Salt and Pepper to taste

Directions

Add the butter and extra virgin olive oil to a large skillet on the stove at medium-high heat. Once the butter is melted, add the shallot. Add a little salt, and let the shallot cook for 1 minute. Then add the mushrooms and thyme. Let them cook for 1 minute. Then add the garlic. Cook for 1 minute, stirring often.

Next add the Port to deglaze the pan (optional). Let that simmer for 1 minute. Add the half & half. Reduce the heat to medium. Let that simmer for 2 minutes. Add the gorgonzola crumbles. Stir gently to melt the cheese into the sauce. Start adding the milk about a 1/4 cup at a time, letting the soup reduce and thicken up.

Once all the milk is added transfer the soup to a slow cooker to continue cooking on low for 1 hour. This step will change the caloric content, and create a thicker, richer soup. (Optional)

Serving Size: 3/4 cup

Number of Servings: 4

Nutrition Information/Serving:

Calories: 276
Fat: 20g
Carbohydrates: 12g
Protein: 11g

Filet with Prosciutto Wrapped Asparagus
4 oz. Filet Mignon, Grilled 202
1/2 cup Simply Potatoes Garlic Mashed Potatoes 104
Prosciutto Wrapped Asparagus w/Balsamic Glaze, recipe follows (about 5 spears) 103
Total Calories 409

Prosciutto Wrapped Asparagus w/Balsamic Glaze

Ingredients
1 bunch of asparagus
1/2 tsp extra virgin olive oil
1 to 2 Tbsp. balsamic glaze to taste (you can find it at specialty Italian stores if your grocer doesn't carry it.)
Fresh ground sea salt & pepper
4oz. of Prosciutto

Directions
Preheat the oven to 425 degrees.

In a large bowl, toss the spears in the oil and the balsamic glaze. Season with salt and pepper. Be careful not to overdo the salt. The prosciutto is salty. Let the seasoned asparagus sit for few minutes.

Cut the prosciutto in half width-wise. Wrap each piece of asparagus with half a slice of the prosciutto.

Lay the spears in a single layer on a medium nonstick baking sheet. Bake them for 4 minutes, flip them, and continue baking until the spears are crisp-tender, 3 to 6 minutes depending on thickness. Season to taste. Serve immediately.

Number of Servings: 4

Nutrition Information/Serving:

Calories: 103
Fat: 6g
Carbohydrates: 6g
Protein: 7g

Grilled Sirloin & Cheesy Mashed Cauliflower
4 oz. Lean Sirloin, Grilled 212
½ cup Loaded Mashed Cauliflower, recipe follows 143
1 cup Green Beans, Steamed 44
Total Calories 399

Loaded Mashed Cauliflower

Ingredients
1 Large Head of Cauliflower, chopped
2 Tbsp. Whipped Cream Cheese
1 Tbsp. Butter with Olive Oil spread
1/2 cup Cheddar Cheese, Shredded
1 tsp. Minced Garlic, from a jar (optional)
Salt to taste

For Garnishing
6 slices of bacon, cooked crisp
2 scallions, chopped
1/4 cup Cheddar Cheese, shredded

Directions
Steam cauliflower 8-12 minutes or until fork tender. Mix it up in a food processor adding a little at a time in batches. Add cream cheese, butter, 1/2 cup cheddar, garlic, and salt. Mix it up again. Transfer to a serving bowl. Garnish with the remaining ingredients.

Serving Size: 1/2 cup

Number of Servings: 6

Nutrition Information/Serving:

Calories: 143
Fat: 9g
Total Carbs: 8g
Protein: 9g

Pork

BBQ Pork Chop, Fries & Jalapeno Cole Slaw
1 BBQ Pork Chop, recipe follows 373
½ cup Jalapeno Cole Slaw, recipe follows 37
Alexia Sweet Potato Fries, baked (12 pieces) 140
Total Calories 550

Cast Iron BBQ Pork Chops

Ingredients
2 thick-cut bone in pork chops
Meat tenderizer
Salt
Pepper
½ cup All-purpose Flour
¼ tsp. Crushed red pepper flakes
1 Tbsp. Olive oil or Canola Oil
4 Tbsp. Barbecue Sauce

Directions
Preheat the oven to 350 degrees.

Pat each side of pork chops dry with a paper towel. Season each side with a light dusting of meat tenderizer, and season with salt & pepper. Let the pork chops sit a few minutes to come up to room temp.

Season flour with crushed red pepper and spread into a thin layer on a plate.

Flour each side of the pork chops. Fluff the flour mixture with a fork between each side for even coating. This will also make the flour go further without getting clumpy. Discard the remaining flour.

Preheat oiled cast iron skillet on medium high heat. Add 1 tbsp. of olive oil to the pan. Once the pan starts to smoke slightly add the pork chops to the pan. Pan sear each side of the chops 3 minutes.

Top each pork chop with 2 Tbsp. of barbecue sauce.

Transfer the cast iron skillet to the preheated oven. Bake for 8 to 10 minutes on top middle oven rack until fork tender.

For thinner chops decrease cooking time and baking temp.

Serving Size: 1 Pork Chop, 4 oz. of pork

Nutritional Information/Serving:

Calories: 373
Total Fat: 16g
Total Carbs: 27g
Protein: 26g

Jalapeno Cole Slaw

Ingredients
2-3 Jalapenos, minced (about 1/3 cup), seeded and deveined
3 cups green Cabbage, shredded
1/3 cup Red onion, diced
1/4 cup Carrot, shredded
1/4 cup Non-fat Greek yogurt
1/4 cup Light mayo
Juice from 1/2 lime
1/4 tsp. Cumin
1/8 tsp. Smoked Paprika
Salt & pepper to taste
Chopped Fresh Cilantro (garnish before serving, optional)

Directions
Combine the jalapenos, cabbage, red onion, and carrot in a mixing bowl. In a separate mixing bowl combine the yogurt, mayo, lime juice, cumin, and paprika for the dressing. Dress the slaw and serve.

Serving Size: ½ cup

Nutritional Information/Serving:

Calories: 37
Total Fat: 2g
Total Carbs: 4g
Protein: 2g

Sausage & Pepperoni Pita Pizza

Ingredients
1 White or Wheat Pita (6.5" diameter)
7 Pepperoni Slices
2 oz. Pork Sausage
¼ cup Mozzarella, shredded
¼ cup Classico Traditional Pizza Sauce

Directions
Preheat the oven to 350 degrees. Brown the sausage in a skillet and drain off excess grease. Spread the pizza sauce on the pita. Top with the sausage, pepperoni, and cheese. Bake in the oven for 12 to 15 minutes.

Serving Size: 1 pizza

Nutrition Information/Serving:

Calories: 535
Fat: 28g
Carbohydrates: 42g
Protein: 26g

Gluten-Free & Vegetarian

Gluten-Free Spinach Ravioli
Conte's Frozen Gluten-Free Spinach Ravioli, 1.5 servings (6 Ravioli) 405
1/3 cup Crushed Tomatoes, sautéed with garlic and basil 33
1 Tbsp. Parmesan, grated 22
½ cup Cremini Mushrooms, fresh, sliced, sautéed 9
1 Tbsp. Brummel & Brown Spread or use cooking spray, for sauté, 45
Total Calories 514

Gluten-Free Veggie Quesadilla

Ingredients
2 Soft Corn Tortillas
1/4 cup Kuner's Refried Black Beans with Lime Juice
1/4 cup Colby Monterey Jack Cheese, Shredded
1/3 cup Bird's Eye Ultimate Southwest Blend (frozen corn, onion, black bean, and poblano pepper mix)
2 Tbsp. Sour Cream
2 Tbsp. Pico de Gallo
Cooking Spray

Directions
The first step is optional. I spray each side of the tortillas with cooking spray. Then place the tortillas on a cookie sheet. Broil them on high for 1 minute on each side in the oven to soften them.

Next preheat the oven at 350 degrees. Spread the re-fried black beans evenly on each tortilla. Be sure to coat close to the edge of the tortilla.

Next top each tortilla with the Colby Jack cheese. Microwave the frozen Southwest blend for 30 seconds to heat/thaw the vegetables. Drain and add to each tortilla.

Bake each tortilla open-faced in the oven for 10 minutes until the cheese is melted. Next broil them on high for 2 minutes until the cheese is slightly browned for added flavor. Make sure you keep an eye on them so that the tortillas don't burn.

Then flip one tortilla on top of the other and cut it into quarters. Garnish with the sour cream and Pico de Gallo.

Serving Size: 1 quesadilla

Nutrition Information/Serving:

Calories: 350
Fat: 16g
Carbohydrates: 41g
Protein: 14g